NEUROMETHODS ☐ 29

Apoptosis Techniques and Protocols

NEUROMETHODS

Program Editors: Alan A. Boulton and Glen B. Baker

NEUROMETHODS □ 29

Apoptosis Techniques and Protocols

Edited by

Judes Poirier

Douglas Hospital Research Centre, Verdun, Canada

Humana Press ✳ Totowa, New Jersey

For additional copies, pricing for bulk purchases, and/or information about other Humana titles, contact Humana at the above address or at any of the following numbers: Tel.: 201-256-1699; Fax: 201-256-8341; E-mail: humana@mindspring.com

Cover illustration: Figure 2 in "Detection of Apoptotic or Necrotic Death in Neuronal Cells by Morphological, Biochemical, and Molecular Analysis," by Martin Gschwind and Gerda Huber.

Cover design by Patricia F. Cleary.

Photocopy Authorization Policy:
Authorization to photocopy items for internal or personal use, or the internal or personal use of specific clients, is granted by Humana Press Inc., provided that the base fee of US $8.00 per copy, plus US $00.25 per page, is paid directly to the Copyright Clearance Center at 222 Rosewood Drive, Danvers, MA 01923. For those organizations that have been granted a photocopy license from the CCC, a separate system of payment has been arranged and is acceptable to Humana Press Inc. The fee code for users of the Transactional Reporting Service is: [0-89603-415-1/97 $8.00 + $00.25].

ISBN 0-89603-415-1
ISSN 0893-2336
Printed in the United States of America. 10 9 8 7 6 5 4 3 2 1

QH573
.P662
1997

1. Cell death

Preface

After many years of neglect, the study of normal cell death and the so-called programmed cell death has finally gained some needed momentum. Evidence obtained over the last five years indicates that programmed cell death (also referred to as apoptosis) occurs normally in most animal tissues at some well-defined stages of their development and/or maturation. The molecular mechanisms by which it is executed remains unknown. However, key regulatory and metabolic steps have been identified in the apoptotic cascade and a central concept has progressively emerged: Apoptosis appears to occur by default in many different cell types unless suppressed by signals originating from neighboring cells. As Martin Raff noted a few years ago, this molecular cascade probably imposes a form of social control on cell survival and cell death.

Since our understanding of the apoptosis phenomena has grown significantly over the last few years, we have been empowered by recent technological advances to biochemically dissect the key metabolic components of apoptotic and necrotic cascades in normal and injured brains. Moreover, the development of improved histochemical tools has allowed us to better define the fundamental criteria of cell death, and transgenic technology has allowed scientists to test working hypotheses pertaining to the mechanism of action of the so-called "cell death gene." Sophisticated molecular biological tools have also enabled us to determine the key elements of normal and abnormal cell cycles, indicating novel functions for the so-called cell-cycle regulated markers that appear to do much more than just regulate cell division.

The present volume of *Apoptosis Techniques and Protocols* now offers neuroscientists at all levels of experience a combination of theoretical and practical information for understanding and studying apoptosis. Topics include the practical

v

analysis of the concepts of necrosis and apoptosis in the CNS as well as histological, biological, and molecular criteria for investigating apoptosis and programmed cell death. Topics range from cellular and invertebrate to animal and human models of apoptosis in various pathological situations in the brain, including Alzheimer's disease, AIDS, and stroke. Numerous techniques are described for examining the critical steps involved in the apoptotic process. These methods range from PCR analysis of cell-cycle regulated proteins, histochemical analysis of DNA degradation, and DNA laddering analysis, to cytochemical alterations of living cells.

It is our hope that *Apoptosis Techniques and Protocols* will prove useful not only as a technical reference, but also as an introduction to the key notions associated with the phenomena of apoptosis and necrosis.

Judes Poirier

Contents

vii

Contributors

RICHARD ALONSO • *Douglas Hospital Research Centre, Centre for Studies on Aging, Departments of Psychiatry and Medicine, McGill University, Montréal, Canada*

MARIA ANKARCRONA • *Department of Environmental Medicine, Karolinska Institute, Stockholm, Sweden*

UWE BEFFERT • *Douglas Hospital Research Centre, Centre for Studies on Aging, Departments of Psychiatry and Medicine, McGill University, Montréal, Canada*

FLOYD E. BLOOM • *Department of Neuropharmacology, The Scripps Research Institute, La Jolla, CA*

EMANUELA BONFOCO • *Department of Environmental Medicine, Karolinska Institute, Stockholm, Sweden*

PATRICIA BOSKA • *Douglas Hospital Research Centre, Centre for Studies on Aging, Departments of Psychiatry and Medicine, McGill University, Montréal, Canada*

DORIS DEA • *Douglas Hospital Research Centre, Centre for Studies on Aging, Departments of Psychiatry and Medicine, McGill University, Montréal, Canada*

PAUL DESJARDINS • *Neuroscience Research Unit, Hôpital St.-Luc, Montréal, Canada*

STEVEN ESTUS • *Department of Physiology, University of Kentucky, Lexington, KY*

HARALD FRANKOWSKI • *Glaxo Institute for Molecular Biology, Geneva, Switzerland*

KATHRIN D. GEIGER • *Edinger-Institut, Universität Frankfurt, Germany*

MARTIN GSCHWIND • *Pharma Division, Preclinical CNS Research, F. Hoffmann La-Roche Ltd., Basel, Switzerland*

GERDA HUBER • *Preclinical CNS Research, Pharma Division, F. Hoffmann La-Roche Ltd., Basel, Switzerland*

GILBERT JAY • *Department of Virology, Jerome H. Holland Laboratory, Rockville, MD*

LISA AYN KERRIGAN • *Departments of Ophthalmology, Molecular Biology and Genetics, and Neuroscience, Johns Hopkins University School of Medicine, Baltimore, MD*

DIMITRI KRAINC • *Laboratory of Cellular and Molecular Neuroscience, Program in Neuroscience and Children's Hospital, Harvard Medical School, Boston, MA*

FRANK M. LAFERLA • *Department of Virology, Jerome H. Holland Laboratory, Rockville, MD*

STÉPHANE LEDOUX • *Neuroscience Research Unit, Hôpital St.-Luc, Montréal, Canada*

STUART A. LIPTON • *Laboratory of Cellular and Molecular Neuroscience, Program in Neuroscience and Children's Hospital, Harvard Medical School, Boston, MA*

THOMAS J. MAHALIK • *Department of Cellular and Structural Biology, University of Colorado Health Sciences Center, Denver, CO*

ISABELLE MARTINOU • *Glaxo Institute for Molecular Biology, Geneva, Switzerland*

JEAN-CLAUDE MARTINOU • *Glaxo Institute for Molecular Biology, Geneva, Switzerland*

DENIS MICHEL • *Laboratoire de Biologie Moléculaire, Campus de Beaulieu, Université de Rennes, France*

MARC MISSOTTEN • *Glaxo Institute for Molecular Biology, Geneva, Switzerland*

EMMANUEL MOYSE • *Laboratoire de Physiologie Neurosensorielle, CNRS-Université Claude Bernard, Villeurbanne, France*

PIERLUIGI NICOTERA • *Department of Environmental Medicine, Karolinska Institute, Stockholm, Sweden; Faculty of Biology, University of Konstanz, Germany*

DAYAN O'DONNELL • *Centre for Studies on Aging, Departments of Psychiatry and Medicine, Douglas Hospital Research Centre, McGill University, Montréal, Canada*

GREGORY P. OWENS • *Department of Neurology, University of Colorado Health Sciences Center, Denver, CO*

STEVEN M. PAUL • *Departments of Pharmacology and Toxicology and Psychiatry, Indiana University School of Medicine, Indianapolis, IN; Lilly Research Laboratories, Eli Lilly and Company, Indianapolis, IN*

JUDES POIRIER • *Centre for Studies on Aging, Departments of Psychiatry and Medicine, Douglas Hospital Research Centre, McGill University, Montréal, Canada*

RÉMY SADOUL • *Glaxo Institute for Molecular Biology, Geneva, Switzerland*

SHAHIN SAKHI • *Department of Neurology, University of Southern California School of Medicine, Los Angeles, CA*

NORA E. SARVETNICK • *Department of Neuropharmacology, The Scripps Research Institute, La Jolla, CA*

STEVEN S. SCHREIBER • *Department of Neurology, University of Southern California School of Medicine, Los Angeles, CA*

MALCOLM WOOD • *Department of Cellular and Structural Biology, University of Colorado Health Sciences Center, Denver, CO*

GUANG-MEI YAN • *Department of Pharmacology and Toxicology, Indiana University School of Medicine, Indianapolis, IN; Lilly Research Laboratories, Eli Lilly and Company, Indianapolis, IN*

DONALD J. ZACK • *Departments of Ophthalmology, Molecular Biology and Genetics, and Neuroscience, Johns Hopkins University School of Medicine, Baltimore, MD*

Gene Tools
to Study Neuronal Apoptosis

Isabelle Martinou, Harald Frankowski,
Marc Missotten, Remy Sadoul,
and Jean-Claude Martinou

1. Introduction

Naturally occurring cell death (NOCD) has been recognized for many years as a critical phase in the development of the nervous system (Hamburger and Levi-Montalcini, 1949; Oppenheim, 1991). During this process, immature neurons undergo an active process of cell death, probably because they receive insufficient quantities of trophic factors from their target cells. Active cell death implies a molecular program of cellular-self-destruction and is therefore often called programmed cell death (PCD) (Schwartz and Osborne, 1993). Diverse morphological types of PCD have been described, with apoptosis being the most commonly encountered (Kerr et al., 1972; Clarke, 1990). After the NOCD period, neuronal apoptosis is considered to be pathological and is found to be implicated in clinical outcomes, such as Alzheimer's disease, Parkinson's disease, or Huntington's disease. It is also observed in acute stresses, such as ischemia. The goal of our laboratory is to identify the molecular mechanisms that underlie PCD in neurons. In this article, we describe the technical approaches undertaken by our laboratory over the last few years to reach this goal.

From: *Neuromethods, Vol. 29: Apoptosis Techniques and Protocols*
Ed: J. Poirier Humana Press Inc.

2. Culture of Sympathetic Neurons as an In Vitro Model System of Neuronal Apoptosis

One of the best documented examples of developmental neuronal death in vertebrates is the demise of 30–50% of the sensory and sympathetic neurons, that depend on nerve growth factor (NGF) for survival (Levi-Montalcini and Brooker, 1960; Thoenen et al., 1987). The type of death triggered by NGF deprivation in vivo can be reproduced in culture. We use sympathetic neurons from rat cervical ganglia that we can maintain in culture for several weeks in the presence of NGF. If NGF is withdrawn from the culture medium, neurons undergo an active death that requires RNA and protein synthesis (Martin et al., 1988; Deckwerth and Johnson, 1993). During PCD, first the cell bodies shrink, then the neurites disintegrate. One of the first morphological signs that can be observed after Hoechst staining is the condensation of the nucleus.

2.1. Microinjection of cDNAs Encoding Diverse Proteins in Sympathetic Neurons

To overexpress different proteins in sympathetic neurons, we microinject DNAs encoding proteins of interest directly into the nucleus. We have found that cytoplasmic injections lead to unefficient transfection. The cDNAs are inserted in an expression vector under the control of a viral promoter. We noticed that cytomegalovirus (CMV) and respiratory syncyalvirus (RSV) promoters are the most potent whereas SV40 promoters give lower expression. For reasons that are unclear, identical promoters confer different levels of expression according to the plasmid vector in which they have been inserted. Microinjection presents several advantages compared to DNA transfer by viruses, the other alternative to transfect efficiently neurons: DNA constructs for microinjection experiments are easy to prepare; and efficacy of transfection can be 100% as all injections can be successful if monitored under fluorescent microscope when a fluorescent dye (Dextran-FITC, for example) has been added to the DNA solution. The disadvantage of this technique is the limited number of neurons that can be microinjected, which impairs biochemical studies of microinjected neurons. Another problem encountered with this technique, as well as with the use of viruses, is associated to the cell system itself. As already mentioned, sympathetic neurons can be protected from NGF deprivation by protein synthesis inhibitors. Therefore, anything that causes a decrease in the overall protein synthesis will protect cells. This may explain why injection of high quantities of DNA that lead to very robust expression of any protein (β-galactosidase, for example) has a rescuing effect. To avoid this problem, we microinject solution at low DNA concentration (0.1–0.05 μg/μL). Moreover, in all experiments, a neutral protein (β-galactosidase) is used as a control. Injection *per se* has no significant effect on neuronal survival.

2.1.1. Proteins that Rescue Sympathetic Neurons from NGF Deprivation

The first protein that was identified as an antidote to neuronal death following NGF deprivation is the bcl-2 protooncogene. Bcl-2 was identified at the chromosomal breakpoint of t(14;18), which constitutes the most common translocation in human lymphoid malignancy (Tsujimoto, 1984). Bcl-2 favors malignancy not by acting on proliferation *per se*, but by blocking programmed cell death. Indeed bcl-2 was first shown to block death of hematopoietic cells induced by withdrawal of IL-3 and IL-4 (Hockenberry et al., 1990). We have microinjected sympathetic neurons with an expression vector containing the cDNA encoding bcl-2. Neurons overexpressing bcl-2 were able to survive for up to 7 d of culture in the absence of NGF, whereas all of the mock-injected neurons died whithin 2–3 d (Garcia et al., 1992). Since then Allsopp et al. (1993) and Mah et al. (1993) have also shown that other neurons that depend on brain-derived neurotrophic factor or neurotrophin 3 for survival can also be protected by bcl-2. Surprisingly, bcl-2 had no effect on ciliary neurons that depend on ciliary neurotrophic factor (CNTF) for survival (Allsopp et al., 1993). Together, these observations suggest that bcl-2-sensitive and bcl-2-insensitive cell death pathways coexist during development of the nervous system. The apparent selectivity of bcl-2 action has its parallel in the hematopoietic system where, in contrast to observations with IL-3- or IL-4-dependent cells, bcl-2 is ineffective in preventing T-cell negative selection against super-antigen or apoptosis in hematopoietic cell lines following IL-6 or IL-2 deprivation (Nunez et al., 1991). However, these observations do not exclude the possibility that the CNTF removal in ciliary neurons or IL-6 and IL-2 deprivation in T-cells could initiate the death program downstream of bcl-2.

Bcl-2 is the prototype of a family whose members can be divided in two subgroups: antiapoptotic proteins bcl-2, bcl-x being the most important) and proapoptotic proteins (Bax, Bak, and Bad).

The bcl-x gene encodes two proteins, bcl-xl and bcl-xs, which are the products of alternative splicing. The longest protein, bclxl is similar in size and predicted structure to bcl-2. Like bcl-2, bcl-xl blocks cell death induced by IL-3 deprivation in lymphocytes (Boise et al., 1993). We found that Bcl-xl is expressed in the nervous system throughout development, whereas Bcl-2 is mainly expressed during early phases of development. Bcl-xl is as efficient as Bcl-2 in blocking PCD in sympathetic neurons (Frankowski et al., 1995; Gonzalez-Garcia et al., 1995).

Bcl-xs, which lacks domains BH1 and BH2 of bcl-2, was shown to counteract the death blocking effect of both bcl-2 and bcl-xl (Boise et al., 1993; Martinou et al., 1995). Bcl-xs was not detected in the rat nervous system (Frankowski et al., 1995).

Two viral proteins, E1B19kD from adenovirus and p35 from baculovirus, were also found to promote survival of sympathetic neurons in the absence of neurotrophic factors (Martinou et al., 1995). E1B19kD shows limited structural homology with bcl-2. p35 was recently found to be an inhibitor of proteases of the interleukin-1β converting enzyme (ICE) family.

Table 1

List of Proteins Overexpressed in Sympathetic Neurons
Cultured in the Presence or Absence of NGF

	Prevents death	Triggers death
bcl-2	+	−
bcl-xL	+	−
bcl-xs	−	−
E1B19K	+	−
p 35	+	−
CrmA	+	−
Bak	−	+
Bax	−	+
Nedd-2	−	+
ICE	−	+/−
CPP 32	−	+/−
Cyclin D1	−	−
WAF1/p 21	−	−
cdc 2	−	−
p 53	−	−
E1A	−	−
E1B55K	−	−
Retinoblastoma gene	−	−
TIA 40	−	−
Ced 4	−	−

We have also tested other proteins whose functions suggested that they could be implicated in cell death. These proteins are listed in Table 1.

2.1.2. Proteins That Trigger Cell Death in Sympathetic Neurons Cultured in the Presence of NGF

We have shown that both Bax and Bak can not only accelerate the kinetics of death of sympathetic neurons after NGF deprivation, but also trigger cell death in neurons cultured in the presence of NGF, that is in the absence of any apparent cell death stimulus (Sadoul et al., submitted).

Studies with the nematode *Caenorhabditis elegans* have identified genes involved in programmed cell death. Two genes, ced-3 and ced-4, are required for normal death to occur (Yuan and Horwitz, 1990). Ced-3 displays structural homologies with ICE, the cysteine protease that converts proIL-1β into active IL-1β (Yuan et al., 1993). A killing function for ICE was suggested by the finding that mammalian fibroblasts and sensory neurons undergo apoptosis after transfection with ICE (Miura et al., 1993). In favor of this hypothesis, Crm-A, a cowpox virus serpin that inhibits ICE (Ray et al., 1992) rescue sensory neurons from NGF deprivation (Gagliardini et al., 1994). These observations suggest that ICE or a related protease plays an important role in apoptosis. ICE and Ced 3 are the founding members of a large family of proteases, including Nedd-2/Ich-1, Ich-2, Mch2, CPP32, ICE-Lap3, and TX (for review, *see* Kumar, 1995; Yuan, 1995). All are synthesized as proenzymes and cleaved at aspartate residues into two subunits of approx 20 and 10 kDa. Several members of this family, including Nedd-2, ICE, and CPP32, have been overexpressed as proenzymes in sympathetic neurons cultured in the presence of NGF. Nedd-2, and to a lesser degree ICE, were found to trigger PCD.

3. Transgenic Mice in the Study of Neuronal Apoptosis

3.1. Bcl-2 Protects Neurons During NOCD

The temporal and spatial pattern of bcl-2 expression in the developing nervous system is consistent with bcl-2 regulating neuronal selection during development (Merry et al., 1994). To test if bcl-2 is capable of protecting neurons from naturally occurring cell death (NOCD), we have generated transgenic mice in which bcl-2 expression was under control of the neuron-specific enolase promoter (Martinou et al., 1994; Dubois-Dauphin et al., 1994). We used a 1.8-kb 5'-flanking region of the rat NSE gene previously shown by Forss-Petter et al. (1990) to drive expression of a reporter gene specifically in neurons. We added to our construct the SV40 T intron at the 3' of bcl-2 cDNA to enhance gene expression. In these mice, a sustained bcl-2 overexpression was detected in most neurons from the onset of the developmental period of NOCD. Unexpectedly, we noted that oligodendrocytes also expressed the transgene. The reason for this ectopic expression is unclear. One possibility is that the presence of the SV40 T intron might influence the promoter activity.

A detailed analysis of the nervous system of the transgenic mice led to the striking observation that different brain regions contain 40–60% more neurons than normal (facial nucleus, ganglion cells of the retina, Martinou et al., 1994; Burne et al., 1995; Purkinje cells, olivary neurons, Zanjani et al., 1996). This demonstrates that at least some neurons use death-pathways that can be blocked by bcl-2 and suggest that the differential regulation of bcl-2 expression could underlie neuronal selection. It will now be of interest to determine whether epigenetic factors regulating NOCD, such as electrical activity, neurotrophic factors, cell-cell, or cell-matrix interactions, influence bcl-2 expression. Since mice lacking bcl-2 were not reported to have any obvious neurological phenotype (Veis et al., 1993), a definite proof that endogenous bcl-2 expression regulates neuronal selection awaits a precise analysis of neuronal systems in these animals. In contrast to Bcl-2, Bcl-xL was found to be required for normal development as mice lacking Bcl-x gene die at E12 due to a massive loss of neurons (Katayama et al., 1995).

3.2. Bcl-2 Protects Neurons Under Pathological Circumstances Induced Experimentally

We have tested whether bcl-2 could protect facial motor neurons from axotomy, a paradigm for motor-neurodegenerative disease. In newborn rodents, transection of the facial nerve normally leads to rapid degeneration of the axotomized motor neurons. In bcl-2 overexpressing transgenic animals, axotomized neurons did not degenerate. Not only were the cell bodies rescued, but also the proximal part of the nerve stayed intact, indicating that bcl-2 overexpression maintained integrity of the damaged axons (Dubois-Dauphin et al., 1994).

We have also used adult transgenic mice to test for survival of cortical neurons after ischemia following permanent middle cerebral artery occlusion (MCAO). MCAO is regarded as a experimental correlate to human stroke. Interestingly, we found that after 7 d of occlusion, there was a 40% reduction in ischemic volume (an index of neuronal death) in transgenic mice as compared to wild-type animals (Martinou et al., 1994). Recent reports have demonstrated that DNA fragmentation occurs in brain after ischemic insult and that protein synthesis inhibitors reduce hippocampal neuronal loss induced by ischemia (Sei et al., 1994; MacManus et al., 1994; Goto et al., 1990; Shigeno et al., 1990). These observations strongly suggest a role for apoptotic death following ischemic damage. The protecting activity of bcl-2 in ischemia that we have observed may be another argument in favor of an apoptotic component to ischemia.

4. Conclusion

The mechanisms by which Bcl-2 and other members of this family function are still poorly understood. We have evidence that bcl-2 acts upstream of proteases of the ICE family in some pathways that lead to cell death (Estoppey et al., 1996). However, as mentioned here, there are death pathways that clearly escape Bcl-2 control. It is possible that these death pathways are initiated downstream to Bcl-2, perhaps by direct protease activation. In agreement with this hypothesis, it has been shown that FAS transduced apoptosis is prevented by inhibitors of ICE proteases, whereas Bcl-2 provides little protection. It will be interesting to test whether overexpression of ICE protease inhibitors, such as CrmA or p35 in transgenic mice leads to a phenotype different from that of mice overexpressing Bcl-2.

Acknowledgments

We thank Steve Arkinstall, Mike Edgerton, Jonathan Knowles, and Karin Sadoul for reading the manuscript.

References

Allsopp T. E. Wyatt S., Patterson H. F., and Davies A. M. (1993) The protooncogene bcl-2 can selectively rescue neutrophic factor-dependent neurons from apoptosis. *Cell* **73**, 95–307.

Boise L. H., Gonzales–Garcia M., Postema C. E., Ding L., Lindsten T., Turka L. A., Mao X., Nunes G., and Thompson C. B. (1993) bcl-x a bcl-2 related gene that functions as a dominant regulator of apoptotic cell death. *Cell* **74**, 597–608.

Clarke P. G. H. (1990) Developmental cell death: morphological diversity and multiple mechanisms. *Anat. Embronyl.* **181**, 195–213.

Deckwerth T. L. and Johnson E. M. (1993) Temporal analysis of events associated with programmed cell death (apoptosis) of sympathetic neurons deprived of nerve growth factor. *J. Cell Biol.* **123(5)**, 1207–1222.

Dubois-Dauphin M., Frankowski H., Tsujimoto Y., Huarte J., and Martinou. J. C. (1994) Neonatal motor neurons overexpressing the bcl-2 protooncogene in transgenic mice are protected from axotomy-induced cell death. *Proc. Natl. Acad. Sci. USA* **91**, 2459–2463.

Estoppey S., Rodriguez I., Sadoul R., and Martinou J.-C. (1996) Bcl-2 prevents activation of CPP32 cysteine protease and cleavage of poly (ADP-ribose) polymerase and v1-70 kD proteins in staurosporine-mediated apoptosis. *Cell Death Diff.,* in press.

Gagliardini V., Fernandez P. A., Lee R. K. K., Drexler H. C. A., Rotello R. J., Fishman M. C., and Yuan J. (1994) Prevention of vertabrate neuronal death by the crmA gene. *Science* **263**, 826–828.

Garcia I., Martinou I., Tsujimoto Y., and Martinou J. C. (1992) Prevention of programmed cell death of sympathetic neurons by the bcl-2 proto-oncogene. *Science* **258**, 302–304.

Goto K., Ishige A., Sekigushi K., Izuka S., Sugimoto A., Yuzurihara M., Aburada M., Hosoya E., and Kogure K. (1930) Effect of cyclohex-imide on delayed neuronal death in rat hippocampus. *Brain Res.* **534**, 299–302.

Hamburger V. and Levi-Montalcini R. (1949) Proliferation differentiation and degeneration of the spinal ganglia of the chick embryo under normal and experimental conditions. *J. Exp. Zool.* **111**, 457.

Hockenbery D., Nunes G., Milliman C., Schreiber R. D., and Korsmeyer S. J. (1990) bcl-2 is an inner mitochondrial membrane protein that blocks programmed cell death. *Nature* **348**, 334–336.

Hockenbery D. M., Oltvai Z. N., Yin X. M., Milliman C. L., and Korsmeyer S. J. (1993) bcl-2 functions in an antioxidant pathway to prevent apoptosis. *Cell* **75**, 241–251.

Kane D. J., Sarafian T. A., Anton R., Hahn H., Butler Gralla E., Selverstone Valentine J., Ord T., and Bredesen D. E. (1993) bcl-2 inhibition of neural death: decreased generation of reactive oxygen species. *Science* **262**, 1274–1277.

Kerr J. F. R. Wyllie A. H., and Currie A. R. (1972) Apoptosis, a basic biological phenomenon with wide-ranging implications in tissue kinectics. *Br. J. Cancer* **26,** 239–257.

Kumar S. (1995) ICE-like proteases in apoptosis. *Trends Biochem. Sci.* **20,** 198–202.

Levi-Montalcini R. and Booker B. (1960) Destruction of the sympathetic ganglia in mammals by an antiserum to the nerve-growth promoting factor. *Proc. Natl. Acad. Sci. USA* **42,** 384–391.

MacManus J. P., Hill I. E., Huang Z. G., Rasquinha I. Xue D., and Buchan A. M. (1994) DNA damage consistent with apoptosis in transient ischaemic. *Neuro Report* **5,** 493–496.

Mah S. P., Zhong L. T., Liu Y., Roghani A., Edwards R. H., and Bredesen D. E. (1993) The protooncogene bcl-2 inhibits apoptosis in PC12 cells. *J. Neurochem.* **60,** 1183–1186.

Martin D. P., Schmidt R. E., Distefano D. P., Lowry O. H., Carter J. G., and Johnson E. M., Jr. (1988) Inhibitors of protein synthesis and RNA synthesis prevent neuronal cell death caused by nerve growth factor deprivation. *J. Cell. Biol.* **106,** 829–844.

Merry D. E., Veis D. J., Hickey W. F., and Korsmeyer S. J. (1994) bcl-2 protein expression is widespread in the developing nervous system and retained in the adult PNS. *Development* **120,** 301–311.

Miura M., Zhu H., Rotello R., Elartwieg E. A. and Yuan J. (1993) Induction of apoptosis by IL-1b-converting enzyme a mammalian homolog of the *C. elegans* cell death gene ced-3. *Cell* **75,** 653–660.

Mortensen A. M. and Novak R. F. (1992) Dynamic changes in the distribution of the calcium-activated neutral protease in human red blood cells following cellular insult and altered calcium homeostasis. *Toxicol Appl. Pharmacol.* **117,** 180–188.

Motoyama N. Wana F., Roth K. A., Sawa H., Nakayama K., Negishi L., Senju S., Zhang Q., Fuji S., et al. (1995) Massive cell death of immature hematopoietic cells and neurons in bcl-x deficient mice. *Science* **267,** 1506–1510.

Nunez G., Hockenbery D. McDonnell T. J., Sorensen C. M., and Korsmeyer S. J. (1991) bcl-2 maintains B cell memory. *Nature* **353,** 71–73.

Raff M. C., Barres. B. A., Burne. J. F., Coles H. S., Ishizaki Y., and Jacobson M. D. (1993) Programmed cell death and the control of cell survival: lessons from the nervous system. *Science* **262,** 695–700.

Ray C. A., Black R. A., Kronheirm S. R., Greenstreet T. A., Sleath P. R., Salvesen G. S., and Pickup D. (1992) Viral inhibition of inflammation: cowpox virus encodes an inhibitor of the interleukin-b converting enzyme. *Cell* **69,** 597–604.

Schwartz L. M. and Osborne. B. (1993) Programmed cell death, apoptosis and killer genes. *Immunol. Today* **14,** 582–590.

Sei Y., Von Lubitz D. K. J. E., Basile A. S. B., Borner M. M., Lin R. C.-S., Skolnick P., and Fossom L. H. (1994) Internucleosomal DNA fragmentation in gerbil hippocampus following forebrain ischemia. *Neurosci. Lett.* **171**, 179–182.

Sendtner M., Holtmann B., Kolbleck R., Thoenen H., and Barde Y. A. (1992) Brain-derived neurotrophic factor prevents the death of motor neurons in newborn rats after nerve section. *Nature* **360**, 757–759.

Shigeno T., Yamasaki Y., Kato G., Kusaka K., Mima T., Takakura K., Graham D., and Furukawa S. (1990) Reduction of delayed neuronal death by inhibition of protein synthesis. *Neurosci. Lett.* **120**, 117–119.

Thoenen H., Bandtlow C., and Heumann R. (1987) The physiological function of nerve growth factor in the central nervous sytem: comparison with the periphery. *Rev. Physiol. Biochem. Pharmacol.* **109**, 145–178.

Thornberry N. A., Bull H. G., Calayay J. R., Chapman K. T., Howard A. D., Kostura M. J., et al. (1992) A novel heterodimeric cysteine protease is required for interleukin-1b processing in monocytes. *Nature* **356**, 768–774.

Tsujimoto Y. and Croce C. M. (1986) Analysis of the structure transcripts and protein products of bcl-2: the gene involved in human follicular lymphoma *Proc. Natl. Acad. Sci. USA* **83**, 5214–5218.

Veis D. J., Sorenson C. M., Shutter J. R., and Fiorsmeyer S. J. (1993) bcl-2-deficient mice demonstrate fulminant lymphoid apoptosis polycystic kidneys and hypopigmented hair. *Cell* **75**, 229–240.

Wood K. A., Dipasquale B., and Youle R. J. (1993) *In situ* labeling of granule cells for apoptosis-associated DNA fragmentation reveals different mechanisms of cell loss in developing cerebellum. *Neuron* **11**, 621–632.

Yuan J., and Horvitz H. R. (1990) The Caenorhabditis elegans genes ced-3 and ced4 act cell autonomously to cause programmed cell death. *Dev. Biol.* **138**, 33–41.

Yuan J., Shaham S., Ledoux S., Ellis H. M., and Horvitz H. R. (1993) The *C. elegans* cell death gene ced-3 encodes a protein similar to mammalian Interleukin-1b-converting enzyme. *Cell* **75**, 641–652.

Yuan J. (1995) Molecular control of life and death. *Curr. Opinion Cell. Biol.* **7**, 211–214.

Zanjani H. S., Vogel M. W., Delhayebouchaud N., Martinou J. C., and Mariani J. (1996) Increased cerebellar Purkinje cell numbers in mice overexpressing a human bcl-2 transgene. *J. Comp. Neurol.* **374**, 332–341.

Detection of Apoptotic or Necrotic Death in Neuronal Cells by Morphological, Biochemical, and Molecular Analysis

Martin Gschwind and Gerda Huber

1. Introduction

1.1. Neuronal Cell Death: Apoptosis vs Necrosis

During embryogenesis of vertebrates, programmed cell death (or apoptosis) is an important event involved in tissue formation and organogenesis (Ernst, 1926; Glücksmann, 1951; Kerr et al., 1972). In the nervous system, programmed cell death of sensory and motor neurons occurs in embryonic stages, but also maturation of central and peripheral nervous system is accompanied by extensive deletion of supernumerary neurons. Furthermore, neuronal cell death is not only part of normal brain development, it also occurs in neurodegenerative disorders.

In humans the most common form of chronic neurodegeneration is Alzheimer's disease (AD) with neuropathological features, such as amyloid deposits, neurofibrillary tangles, and in particular, selective loss of neurons in the brain (for reviews *see* Katzman and Saitoh, 1991; Selkoe, 1991). The major component of the extracellular amyloid deposits is the 39–43 residue Aβ-peptide (Glenner and Wong, 1984) derived from β-amyloid precursor proteins (β-APPs) by proteolysis (Goldgaber et al., 1987; Kang et al., 1987; Tanzi et al., 1987;

From: *Neuromethods, Vol. 29: Apoptosis Techniques and Protocols*
Ed: J. Poirier Humana Press Inc.

Bendotti et al., 1988). Neuronal degeneration is found around amyloid plaques and it was postulated that Aβ causes neuronal cell death (Tanzi et al., 1989; Selkoe, 1991). Although this was demonstrated in vitro (Yankner et al., 1989; Forloni et al., 1993; Loo et al., 1993; Behl et al., 1994; Gschwind and Huber, 1995), conflicting results exist concerning neuronal cell death in vivo following injection of purified plaque material or synthetic Aβ into animal brains (Emre et al., 1992; Games et al., 1992; Kowall et al., 1992; Stephenson and Clemens, 1992). Increased generation of Aβ (Citron et al., 1992; Cai et al., 1993; Johnston et al., 1994) or a shift toward a 2 residue larger form thereof, $A\beta_{1-42}$ (Suzuki et al., 1994; Tamaoka et al., 1994), is associated with missense mutations in the β-APP gene in some AD families (Chartier-Harlin et al., 1991; Goate et al., 1991; Murrell et al., 1991; Mullan et al., 1992). This "aberrant" load of Aβ peptide in AD brain supports the amyloid cascade hypothesis of Aβ deposits directly causing AD neurodegeneration. However, it is poorly understood how the peptide would induce this effect. Therefore, characterization of Aβ-induced cell death might shed some light on the molecular mechanisms of this highly common form of neurodegeneration.

Cell death can be distinguished morphologically and biochemically into two distinct pathways, necrosis and apoptosis (Wyllie et al., 1980). Necrosis is normally the result of a severe insult resulting in cell damage characterized by rapid breakdown of all membrane systems and disruption of organelles as the whole cell swells and increases in size. Inflammatory responses are usually a consequence of necrotic cell death. In contrast, apoptosis is the result of several well orchestrated events that require RNA and protein synthesis induced by certain stimuli (Cohen and Duke, 1984; Wyllie et al., 1984). Morphological changes seen in cells undergoing apoptosis include condensation and fragmentation of heterochromatin and the formation of apoptotic bodies. This is followed by membrane blebbing and cellular fragmentation, in which most of the organelles remain intact. Whereas, in necrosis, DNA becomes degraded randomly during cell death, internucleosomally fragmented DNA is found at an early stage of apoptosis owing to induced endonuclease activity.

2. Cellular Models of Cell Death

2.1. Cell Cultures

Neuronal cell death can be studied either using primary neuronal cultures or neuronal cell lines. Immortalized cell lines of neuronal origin, such as neuroblastomas have some advantages over primary neuronal cultures in being much easier to cultivate and in not representing a mixture of several cell types which makes certain analyses of cell death more difficult. Thus, various neuronal cell lines should preferably be compared with each other when investigating the effect of a potentially toxic agent, because each cell type might react in its own way. Combined results may then give a unique picture or else may differentiate the findings for in vivo relevance.

Thus, in order to study Aβ-induced cell death, a range of cell types, such as rat pheochromocytoma PC12, mouse neuroblastoma NB_2a, rat neuroblastoma B104, and human neuroblastoma IMR32 cells could be used. These cell lines are best maintained in serum containing medium at moderate density to prevent differentiation. NB_2a and B104 cells can be cultured in Dulbecco's modified Eagle's medium, supplemented with 50 µg/mL gentamicin and 10% fetal calf serum (heat-inactivated) at 37°C, 10% CO_2. The same medium supplemented with additional 5% horse serum is suitable to grow PC12 and IMR32 cells. Stock plates of all cell lines are passaged routinely every 2–3 d onto new polystyrene tissue culture dishes (Falcon, Los Angeles; uncoated). B104 cells have to be trypsinized first for 7 min at 37°C with trypsin-EDTA solution (1X, Gibco-BRL, Gaithersburg, MD), whereas PC12, IMR32, and NB_2a cells can easily be washed off the dishes with fresh culture medium before dividing.

2.2. Induction of Cell Death

For quantitative investigation of neurotoxicity in cell culture, certain precautions need to be taken. First of all, dying cells tend to detach easily from the substratum and, therefore, analysis methods that include washing steps on the substratum detect only the remaining healthy cells. Proper adhesion of cells to the substratum is, thus, very important and weakly adhering cell types can be grown on collagen-coated plastic and glassware instead of on polystyrene dishes. Either precoated culture dishes are used (e.g., Corning, Kleiner AG, Switzerland) or standard plastic and glassware is coated in the following way: Collagen R (0.2%, Serva, Heidelberg, Germany), diluted with sterile water to 60 µg/mL, covers the surfaces at 100 µL/cm^2 and is air dried onto the surface over-night in a laminar flow (6 µg collagen R/cm^2).

The culture medium represents another problem. Although serum containing medium usually provides optimal culture conditions for neuroblastomas, its serum components might interfere when looking at cell death induced by a certain agent. Serum-free media with high glucose can be used instead, although there is the possibility of reduced viability when cells are kept for too long without serum. For example, serum withdrawal for 2 d has absolutely no effect on IMR32, NB$_2$a, and B104 cells, but for PC12 cells at 24 h, up to 20% of the cells start dying owing to serum deprivation (Fig. 1). In this cell line, apoptosis has previously been described after serum withdrawal (Batistatou and Greene, 1991) and, indeed, occasional PC12 cells with typical apoptotic nuclear structure can be found in such cultures. Nevertheless, cells like PC12 can be used to investigate induced cell death if maintained in culture for less than 24 h in serum-free medium. Overall, it is important to determine experimental conditions, in which serum deprivation and exposure time to toxic test agents are as short as possible but long enough to reveal distinct cyto-toxicity of an agent; ideally around 50–70% of cells dying as measured by the lactate dehydrogenase (LDH) assay (*see* Section 4.1.).

For experimental analysis of an exposure time of 24 h, PC12 cells are ideally plated at a density of 4×10^4 cells/cm^2 onto collagen-coated surfaces 18 h prior to treatment. For IMR32, NB$_2$a, and B104 cells a density of 2×10^4 cells/cm^2 is suitable.

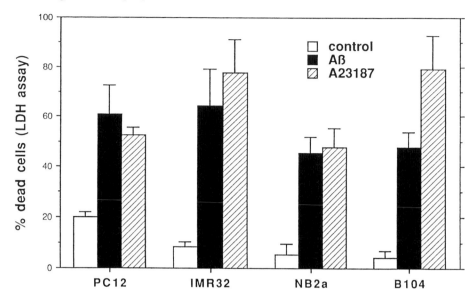

Fig. 1. Quantitation of cell death induced by Aβ and A23187. Different cell types were exposed for 24 h to Aβ (0.5 mg/mL) or A23187 (2 μM) in serum-free medium. Control cultures were cultivated in serum-free medium alone. Cytotoxicity was determined by measuring the LDH activity in the culture supernatant. Values are mean ± SEM (3–6 experiments). Cell death rate in all treated cultures was significantly different from controls ($p < 0.005$, Student's t-test).

After overnight attachment in normal growth medium, the cells are washed once with serum-free medium before exposing them for 24 h in this medium to a potentially toxic agent. In our study Aβ$_{1-42}$, a reverse-sequence peptide (Aβ$_{40-1}$) or the calcium iono-phore A23187 (Calbiochem, La Jolla, CA) were used.

3. Morphological Cell Changes (Phase-Contrast Microscopy)

Cell death in neuronal cultures can be qualitatively monitored using phase-contrast light microscopy. Comparison of cellular morphology of dying cells with healthy untreated ones allows detection of abnormal cellular structures. In IMR32, NB$_2$a, and B104 cells treated with Aβ, these changes included appearance of less new neurites combined with swelling and disintegration of present neurites. Such changes appeared after 5–10 h exposure to 0.5 mg/mL Aβ. Because of the round cell shape and missing neurites in undifferentiated PC12 cells these characteristics were absent in PC12 cells. Degeneration and complete loss of cell bodies resulted in a markedly reduced cell density in all four cell types after 24 h exposure to Aβ. At the same time, total fragmentation of neurites was visible where present (Fig. 2). In contrast to Aβ-treated cells, which disintegrated on the substratum leaving behind cell debris, the same cells exposed to 2 μM of the calcium ionophore A23187 tended to detach completely from culture dish surfaces, leaving nothing behind.

Membrane blebbing, vacuolization, and formation of small apoptotic bodies leading to fragmentation of cells are morphological changes typical for apoptosis with controlled reorganization of cellular compartments. In response to Aβ these changes became evident in PC12, NB_2a, and B104 cells. In contrast, the appearance of Aβ-treated IMR32 cells was different: Neurites and cell bodies were intensely swollen suggesting necrotic cell death with rapid nonspecific breakdown of the whole membrane system. The same morphological differences were seen in PC12, IMR32, and NB_2a cells after 24 h exposure to 2 μM A23187 indicating necrotic cell death in these cell types caused by the calcium ionophore.

4. Biochemical Parameters for Cell Death

4.1. Lactate Dehydrogenase Assay

Dying cells experience extensive breakdown of the cellular membrane system. Thus, in cell culture, the course of cytotoxicity can be easily followed quantitatively by measuring the activity of the cytosolic enzyme lactate dehydrogenase (LDH) in the supernatant. The percentage of dying cells in a culture is represented by LDH activity measured in the supernatant relative to the LDH after complete cell lysis with detergent. This complete membrane disruption can be achieved by addition of 10% Triton X-100 to a final concen-

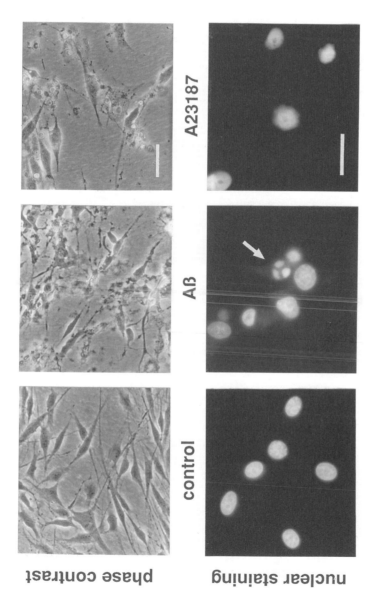

Fig. 2. Morphological changes induced by Aβ and A23187 in B104 cells. Cells were treated with Aβ (0.5 mg/mL) or A23187 (2 μM) in serum-free medium. After 24 h, morphological changes were visualized by phase-contrast microscopy (upper pictures) and by fluorescence microscopy after staining nuclear DNA with Hoechst-33258 (lower pictures). Arrow indicates apoptotic nuclei. Calibration bar is 50 μm for phase-contrast and 25 μm for fluorescence micrographs.

tration of 0.1% directly to the cell cultures. LDH catalyzes the reduction of pyruvate + NADH + H$^+$ to lactate + NAD$^+$. Owing to differences in the absorption spectra of NADH and NAD$^+$, changes in the NADH concentration can be detected at 340 nm. The decrease of OD$_{340}$ thus represents the enzyme activity when using pyruvate as substrate. In the LDH assay, 50-µL samples of cell culture supernatant are assayed in 96-well microtiter plates with 160 µL LDH buffer (90 mM K$_2$HPO$_4$, 15 mM KH$_2$PO$_4$, 1.25 mM sodium pyruvate). After addition of 6 µL NADH solution (13 mM NADH-Na$_2$, 120 mM NaHCO$_3$), decrease of OD$_{340}$ is measured at room temperature in a microplate reader (e.g., Bio-Rad, Hercules, CA). Preceding each measurement, 10 s of vigorous shaking is important in order to mix substrate and enzyme properly. Only conditions of substrate saturation, i.e., linear decay of OD$_{340}$, are suitable to calculate enzyme activity. This needs to be considered, especially when determining the value for 100% cell death, because under these conditions substrate can be used up in as little as 2 min in the assay. The time course of cell toxicity of a test agent can be monitored by analyzing supernatant samples from the same culture at different time points and taking into consideration the step-by-step volume reduction of the remaining culture medium.

The LDH-release measurements for Aβ-induced cell death in PC12, IMR32, NB$_2$a, and B104 cells were done in serum-free medium with high glucose as described before. Control cultures were exposed to the reverse-sequence peptide or maintained in serum-free medium alone. The Aβ clearly was toxic for all four cell types (Gschwind and Huber, 1995). After 24 h treatment with Aβ, depending on cell type, 40–75% dying cells were detected using the LDH assay (Fig. 1). Control cultures showed spontaneous cell death of only 5–10% after the same time in serum-free medium except for PC12 cells, in which 20% of the cells died owing to serum deprivation. Unspecific effects of Aβ could be excluded because there was no difference in viability between cells exposed to the reverse-sequence peptide (Aβ$_{40-1}$) and serum-free medium alone (data not shown). These results demonstrate how the neuroblastoma cell culture systems can ideally be used to show neurotoxic properties of a test agent in vitro.

When dealing with a new potentially neurotoxic agent it is difficult to predict its half maximal effective concentration (EC_{50}) for a certain exposure time, although this is important to get clear results. This problem can be approached in two ways. Either several concentrations are tested for a fixed exposure time or only a few concentrations are examined over a whole time range. The second approach is recommended, especially if the testing material is only available in limited amounts, as the LDH assay allows samples from one cell culture to be measured at different time points in comparison with untreated cultures. Results from this approach not only allow the range for a fixed time EC_{50} to be narrowed down, but are also useful when comparing different agents that might have the same neurotoxic mechanism. For example, Aβ-induced cell death (0.5 mg/mL) was detectable in all cell types with the LDH parameter in as early as 5–10 h, at the same time that the first changes in cellular morphology became obvious by phase-contrast microscopy. In contrast to this, cultures exposed to the calcium ionophore A23187, with the same percentage of dead cells after 24 h as those exposed to Aβ, showed a much faster cytotoxic response. Proposed giant calcium channels formed by Aβ in lipid bilayers (Arispe et al., 1993) hypothesize that Aβ disturbs cellular calcium homeostasis, yet because of the different cell death kinetics it is unlikely that Aβ simply acts as a calcium ionophore like A23187.

4.2. MTT Reduction Assay

Alternatively to the LDH assay, cell viability can also be measured with the 3,(4,5-dimethyl-thiazol-2-yl) 2,5-diphenyl-tetrazolium bromide (MTT) reduction assay (Hansen et al., 1989). In this assay, the tetrazolium salt MTT is converted in intact mitochondria to a colored formazan product that can be detected photometrically after extraction. This method is more sensitive than the LDH assay because already reduced mitochondrial activity of disturbed cells is determined in contrast to membrane leakage of severely damaged cells. But a disadvantage of this method is that only one time-point/cell culture can be measured and long staining and extraction times do not allow cell death to be traced simultaneously during the experiment. Finally, MTT reduction does not necessarily reflect cell death but is a parameter for cellular metabolic activity.

5. Nuclear Morphology and Chromosomal Structure

5.1. Staining of Nuclear DNA with Hoechst-33258

In dying cells, not only overall changes in cellular morphology are visible by phase-contrast microscopy, but also intracellular ultrastructure, i.e., the shape and organization of organelles is affected. For example, the nuclear morphology and chromatin structure are changed drastically during cell death. Additionally, different nuclear events can be associated with apoptotic or necrotic cell death (*see* Section 5.2.). Nuclear shape and chromosomal structure can be visualized by staining nuclear DNA with Hoechst-33258 (Fluka, Buchs, Switzerland).

For this purpose, cells are cultivated on 11 mm Ø glass coverslips coated with collagen (*see* Section 2.2.). It is important to use coated glass coverslips because coated plastic coverslips interfere with the fluorescence microscopy used for detection of the staining. Freshly collagen-coated coverslips stick very hard to the surface on which they have been coated and, thus, have to be detached carefully before placing them in 12-well tissue culture plates for experiments. After exposure of cell cultures to test agents (*see* Section 2.2.), culture medium is aspirated and replaced by 4% paraformaldehyde in PBS. Cells are fixed in this solution for 10 min at room temperature before they are washed once with PBS and stained with 2.5 µg/mL Hoechst-33258 in PBS for 5 min at room temperature. Following the staining procedure, cells are washed once again with PBS before coverslips are mounted with glycerol:PBS (9:1, v/v) on glass slides. Visualization of stained nuclei is performed by fluorescence microscopy, e.g., using a Zeiss axiphot microscope (filter: G365, FT395, LP420) or similar.

5.2. Discrimination Between Necrotic and Apoptotic Nuclei

In dying cells, nuclear morphology changes differ depending on the type of cell death. Nuclei of cells dying in a necrotic way appear swollen, as do whole cell bodies of such cells, and heterochromatin is uniformly dispersed throughout the nuclei. Because of severe membrane damage in necrotic cells, extrusions of nuclear DNA passing the leaky nuclear membrane are often visible. On the other side, in apoptotic cells undergoing a defined program of cellular events, shrinkage of nuclei is observed. In those cells, condensation and fragmentation of heterochromatin is followed by fragmentation of whole nuclei leading to apoptotic bodies containing parts of the former nuclei (Wyllie et al., 1980).

Control cultures of IMR32, NB_2a, and B104 cells maintained in serum-free medium for 24 h revealed intact, round-shaped nuclei with equally dispersed heterochromatin. Only in PC12 cultures occasional nuclei with condensed and fragmented chromatin could be found owing to serum deprivation for 24 h (spontaneous PC12 cell death of up to 20% after 24 h in serum-free medium as determined by the LDH assay, *see* Section 4.2.). Induction of apoptotic cell death owing to serum deprivation was described for this cell type previously (Batistatou and Greene, 1991; Behl et al., 1994).

Following 24 h exposure to Aβ (0.5 mg/mL), condensation and fragmentation of chromatin as well as shrinkage and fragmentation of whole cell nuclei as apoptotic bodies were evident in PC12, NB_2a, and B104 cells after staining of nuclear DNA with Hoechst-33258 (Fig. 2). The most drastic changes could be seen in PC12 cells in which after 11 h of Aβ exposure, many cell nuclei showed these typical apoptotic features and after 24 h, the majority of nuclei were affected. Whereas in Aβ-treated cultures of NB_2a and B104 cells, many apoptotic nuclei were also present, none were found in IMR32 cells. In this cell type, condensed chromatin structures were only seen in nuclei of cells that were clearly undergoing cell division and, thus, not committed to die. In contrast, nuclei of Aβ-treated IMR32 cells were not reduced in size, but looked more amorphous without any defined surface outline, indicating that Aβ-induced cell death in IMR32 cells is necrotic rather than apoptotic.

Morphological nuclear changes apparent after 24 h exposure to the calcium ionophore A23187 (2 μM) clearly differed from those induced by Aβ. Heterochromatin was uniformly packaged in nuclei of all cell types and, like in IMR32 cells incubated with Aβ, the border between cytoplasm and nucleus was very diffuse with extruding nuclear DNA, indicating necrotic cell death in PC12 and B104 cells. In contrast, nuclei of IMR32 and NB_2a cells were round-shaped and strongly reduced in size but without condensed and fragmented chromatin which might represent an early apoptotic event.

6. Internucleosomal DNA Fragmentation in Apoptosis

A hallmark of apoptosis is internucleosomal fragmentation of nuclear DNA, occurring relatively early during cell death as a result of an induced nuclease activity (Cohen and Duke, 1984; Wyllie et al., 1984). This process of specific DNA fragmentation leads to oligonucleosomes of different but defined length, i.e., multiples of 180–200 bp corresponding to DNA content/nucleosome. In contrast, nuclear DNA of necrotic cells remains mainly intact or becomes randomly degraded in severely damaged cells resulting in DNA fragments of heterogeneous length.

For analysis of nuclear internucleosomal DNA fragmentation, cells are grown on 6 cm Ø collagen-coated culture dishes, treated eventually with an experimental toxin and detached from substratum using a cell scraper. The dishes are rinsed once with PBS which is then pooled with the cell suspension. After centrifugation at 250g for 5 min, the cell pellet is washed twice with ice-cold PBS, taken up in 400 µL lysis buffer (100 mM Tris-HCl, pH 8.0, 10 mM EDTA, 0.5% n-lauroylsarcosine, 0.5 mg/mL proteinase K) and incubated at 56°C. After 1.5 h RNase A is added to a final concentration of 0.25 mg/mL and the incubation continued for 10 h. The cell lysates are then extracted twice with equilibrated phenol and twice with isoamylalcohol:chloroform (1:24, v/v). Out of the aqueous phase, DNA is precipitated with 1/10 vol of 3M sodium acetate and 2 vol ethanol at –20°C. The precipitates are washed once with 70% ethanol and resuspended in 30 µL 10 mM Tris-HCl, pH 8.0, 1 mM EDTA. Residual RNA is digested by a second treatment with RNase A (0.25 mg/mL) for 2 h at 37°C before 20 µL of each sample are mixed with 4 µL 40% sucrose and loaded onto 2% agarose gels. Sample buffer without bromphenol blue (i.e., 40% sucrose) should be used to increase visibility in the low molecular range of the gels for better detection of the lowest faint bands of a possible DNA ladder. Gels are run for 2 h at 70 V in electrophoresis buffer (40 mM Tris-acetate pH 8.0, 1 mM EDTA) before DNA is stained with 2 µg/mL ethidium bromide in electrophoresis buffer for 45 min. Gels are destained with 1 mM MgSO$_4$ for 30 min to remove unbound ethidium bromide before photographing under UV light.

After agarose gel electrophoresis of extracted cellular DNA, apoptotic cell death is revealed by the appearance of a typical 180–200 bp DNA ladder. Individual bands of the ladder represent oligonucleosomes of different length produced by the internucleosomal cleavage of nuclear DNA. This laddering is usually not found when looking at DNA from intact cells or cells killed by necrosis that contain only high molecular weight DNA or a smear of randomly degraded DNA.

The Aβ was found to induce apoptotic cell death in PC12, NB$_2$a, and B104 cells but not in IMR32 cells with respect to nuclear structure (*see* Section 5.2.). In order to see whether these findings correlate with internucleosomal fragmentation in nuclei with apoptotic morphology, Aβ-treated cells were examined for the presence of typical DNA ladders by agarose gel electrophoresis. DNA extracted from PC12, NB$_2$a, and B104 cells after 24 h exposure to Aβ was clearly

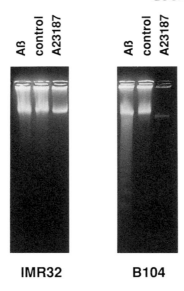

Fig. 3. Molecular structure of nuclear DNA from dead cells. IMR32 and B104 cells were exposed for 24 h to Aβ (0.5 mg/mL) or A23187 (2 μM) in serum-free medium (control cultures in serum-free medium alone). After agarose gel electrophoresis, only Aβ-treated B104 cells show typical apoptotic laddering of internucleosomally fragmented DNA.

internucleosomally fragmented as judged by the DNA laddering (Fig. 3). This was already visible after 11 h in PC12 cells where also the earliest and most dramatic changes in nuclear structure were seen. In Aβ-treated IMR32 cultures, where in contrast to the other cell types no apoptotic nuclear changes were observed, also no DNA fragmentation was detected even after 24 h when the majority of cells had died. Only DNA from IMR32 cells showed no DNA laddering after death by Aβ, i.e., the results were consistent with the morphological changes observed in the different cell types. Thus, not only morphological, but also molecular parameters indicate a more necrotic degeneration in IMR32 cells treated with Aβ, whereas under the same conditions in the other three cell types, apoptosis is induced.

Absence of internucleosomal DNA fragmentation and nonapoptotic nuclear structure in calcium ionophore-treated PC12, IMR32, and B104 cells clearly show calcium influx-dependent necrosis in these cell types. Interestingly, in NB_2a cells, internucleosomal DNA fragmentation occurred after 24 h exposure to A23187, yet no condensed, fragmented chromatin was visible at this time point. However, nuclei of these cells were strongly reduced in size which is a known early step of apoptosis. This suggests that increase in intracellular calcium may cause apoptosis in certain cell types, such as NB_2a cells, although it more frequently induces necrosis. Out of calcium ionophore A23187-treated cultures generally less DNA could be extracted, probably owing to the fact that following rapid cell death complete cellular disintegration occurs.

In control cultures of PC12, IMR32, NB_2a, and B104 cells kept in serum-free medium for 24 h, only intact high molecular weight DNA was found. Remarkably, this included DNA derived from PC12 cells where owing to serum deprivation for 24 h, up to 20% cell death was measured by the LDH assay (*see* Section 4.2.) and, occasionally, few nuclei with apoptotic characteristics were microscopically observed over a large background of nonapoptotic cells (*see* Section 5.2.). Thus, with this protocol, internucleosomal fragmentation in programmed cell death is not detectable by DNA laddering when only a small fraction of cells in a culture is affected. This might be a problem for analyzing primary cultures if only an underrepresented cell type dies in an apoptotic way.

7. Conclusions

Neurotoxicity can be investigated most easily in vitro using tissue culture systems. On one hand, primary neuronal cultures share the complexity of the in vivo situation but have the disadvantage of representing a mixture of several different cell types which not all may react in the same way. Thus, comparison of different individually treated neuroblastoma lines allows more accurate discrimination between apoptotic and necrotic cell death induced by a toxic stimulus depending on the cell type. Application of most protocols described here is therefore, best suitable for pure cultures. Detection of internucleosomal DNA fragmentation by DNA laddering analysis might be especially problematic if only a subpopulation of a mixed culture undergoes apoptosis following a certain stimulus. However, in this case apoptosis can still be detected by microscopic analysis of nuclear DNA stained with Hoechst-33258. Individual cells with condensed and fragmented chromatin and/or apoptotic bodies have to be characterized further to compare their cell type with the rest of the culture. Finally, as shown by this comparison, preferably combinations of different test methods and culture systems should be applied whenever possible in order to obtain a most complete view on the action of a cell-toxic agent.

Acknowledgment

Rat pheochromocytoma PC12 cells were obtained from C. Hertel (F. Hoffmann-La Roche, Basel), neuroblastoma NB_2a and B104 cells from D. Monard (Friedrich Miescher Institute, Basel), and neuroblastoma IMR32 from American Type Cell Culture Collection. The authors thank H. Döbeli and T. Vorherr (F. Hoffmann-La Roche, Basel) for providing β-amyloid peptides. We are also very grateful to J. Kemp and Ch. Köhler for critical reading of the manuscript.

References

Arispe N., Pollard H. B., and Rojas E. (1993) Giant multilevel cation channels formed by Alzheimer disease amyloid beta-protein [A beta P-(1-40)] in bilayer membranes. *Proc. Natl. Acad. Sci. USA* **90,** 10,573–10,577.

Batistatou A. and Greene L. A. (1991) Aurintricarboxylic acid rescues PC12 cells and sympathetic neurons from cell death caused by nerve growth factor deprivation: correlation with suppression of endonuclease activity. *J. Cell Biol.* **115,** 461–471.

Behl C., Davis J. B., Klier F. G., and Schubert D. (1994) Amyloid β peptide induces necrosis rather than apoptosis. *Brain Res.* **645,** 253–264.

Bendotti C., Forloni G. L., Morgan R. A., O'Hara B. F., Oster-Granite M. L., Reeves R. H., Gearhart J. D., and Coyle J. T. (1988) Neuroanatomical localization and quantification of amyloid precursor protein mRNA by *in situ* hybridization in the brains of normal, aneuploid, and lesioned mice. *Proc. Natl. Acad. Sci. USA* **85,** 3628–3632.

Cai X. D., Golde T. E., and Younkin S. G. (1993) Release of excess amyloid beta protein from a mutant amyloid β protein precursor. *Science* **259**, 514–516.

Chartier-Harlin M. C., Crawford F., Houlden H., Warren A., Hughes D., Fidani L., Goate A., Rossor M., Roques P., Hardy J., and Mullan M. (1991) Early-onset Alzheimer's disease caused by mutations at codon 717 of the beta-amyloid precursor protein gene. *Nature* **353**, 844–846.

Citron M., Oltersdorf T., Haass C., McConlogue L., Hung A. Y., Seubert P., Vigo-Pelfrey C., Lieberburg I., and Selkoe D. J. (1992) Mutation of the beta-amyloid precursor protein in familial Alzheimer's disease increases beta-protein production. *Nature* **360**, 672–674.

Cohen J. J. and Duke R. C. (1984) Glucocorticoid activation of a calcium-dependent endonuclease in thymocyte nuclei leads to cell death. *J. Immunol.* **132**, 38–42.

Emre M., Geula C., Ransil B. J., and Mesulam M. M. (1992) The acute neurotoxicity and effects upon cholinergic axons of intracerebrally injected beta-amyloid in the rat brain. *Neurobiol. Aging* **13**, 553–559.

Ernst M. (1926) Über Untergang von Zellen während der normalen Entwicklung bei Wirbeltieren. *Z. Anat. Entwicklungsgesch.* **79**, 228–262.

Forloni G., Chiesa R., Smiroldo S., Verga L., Salmona M., Tagliavini F., and Angeretti N. (1993) Apoptosis mediated neurotoxicity induced by chronic application of beta amyloid fragment 25–35. *Neuroreport* **4**, 523–526.

Games D., Khan K. M., Soriano F. G., Keim P. S., Davis D. L., Bryant K., and Lieberburg I. (1992) Lack of Alzheimer pathology after beta-amyloid protein injections in rat brain. *Neurobiol. Aging* **13**, 569–576.

Glenner G. G. and Wong C. W. (1984) Alzheimer's disease: initial report of the purification and characterization of a novel cerebrovascular amyloid protein. *Biochem. Biophys. Res. Commun.* **120**, 885–890.

Glücksmann A. (1951) Cell death in normal vertebrate ontogeny. *Biol. Rev.* **26**, 59–86.

Goate A., Chartier-Harlin M. C., Mullan M., Brown J., Crawford F., Fidani L., Giuffra L., Haynes A., Irving N., James L., Mant R., Newton P., Rooke K., Roques P., Talbot C., Pericak-Vance M., Roses A., Williamson R., Rossor M., Owen M., and Hardy J. (1991) Segregation of a missense mutation in the amyloid precursor protein gene with familial Alzheimer's disease. *Nature* **349**, 704–706.

Goldgaber D., Lerman M. I., McBride O. W., Saffiotti U., and Gajdusek D. C. (1987) Characterization and chromosomal localization of a cDNA encoding brain amyloid of Alzheimer's disease. *Science* **235**, 877–880.

Gschwind M. and Huber G. (1995) Apoptotic cell death induced by β-amyloid (1-42) peptide is cell type dependent. *J. Neurochem.* **65**, 292–300.

Hansen M. B., Nielsen S. E., and Berg K. (1989) Re-examination and further development of a precise and rapid dye method for measuring cell growth/cell kill. *J. Immunol. Methods* **119**, 203–210.

Johnston J. A., Cowburn R. F., Norgren S., Wiehager B., Venizelos N., Winbald B., Vigo-Pelfrey C., Schenk D., Lannfelt L., and O'Neill C. (1994) Increased β-amyloid release and levels of amyloid precursor protein (APP) in fibroblast cell lines from family members with the Swedish Alzheimer's disease APP670/671 mutation. *FEBS Lett.* **354**, 274–278.

Kang J., Lemaire H. G., Unterbeck A., Salbaum J. M., Masters C. L., Grzeschik K. H., Multhaup G., Beyreuther K., and Muller-Hill B. (1987) The precursor of Alzheimer's disease amyloid A4 protein resembles a cell-surface receptor. *Nature* **325**, 733–736.

Katzman R. and Saitoh T. (1991) Advances in Alzheimer's disease. *FASEB J.* **5**, 278–286.

Kerr J. F. R., Wyllie A. H., and Currie A. R. (1972) Apoptosis: a basic biological phenomenon with wideranging implications in tissue kinetics. *Br. J. Cancer* **26**, 239–257.

Kowall N. W., McKee A. C., Yankner B. A., and Beal M. F. (1992) In vivo neurotoxicity of beta-amyloid [beta(1-40)] and the beta(25-35) fragment. *Neurobiol. Aging* **13**, 537–542.

Loo D. T., Copani A., Pike C. J., Whittemore E. R., Walencewicz A. J., and Cotman C. W. (1993) Apoptosis is induced by beta-amyloid in cultured central nervous system neurons. *Proc. Natl. Acad. Sci. USA* **90**, 7951–7955.

Mullan M., Crawford F., Axelman K., Houlden H., Lilius L., Winbald B., and Lannfelt L. (1992) A pathogenic mutation for probable Alzheimer's disease in the APP gene at the N-terminus of β-amyloid. *Nat. Genet.* **1**, 345–347.

Murrell J., Farlow M., Ghetti B., and Benson M. D. (1991) A mutation in the amyloid precursor protein associated with hereditary Alzheimer's disease. *Science* **254**, 97–99.

Selkoe D. J. (1991) The molecular pathology of Alzheimer's disease. *Neuron* **6**, 487–498.

Stephenson D. T. and Clemens J. A. (1992) In vivo effects of beta-amyloid implants in rodents: lack of potentiation of damage associated with transient global forebrain ischemia. *Brain Res.* **586**, 235–246.

Suzuki N., Cheung T. T., Cai X. D., Odaka A., Otvos L., Eckman C., Golde T. E., and Younkin S. G. (1994) An increased percentage of long amyloid beta protein secreted by familial amyloid beta protein precursor (beta APP717) mutants. *Science* **264**, 1336–1340.

Tamaoka A., Odaka A., Ishibashi Y., Usami M., Sahara N., Suzuki N., Nukina N., Mizusawa H., Shoji S., Kanazawa I., and Mori H. (1994) APP717 Missense mutation affects the ratio of amyloid β protein species (Aβ1-42/43 and Aβ1-40) in familial Alzheimer's disease brain. *J. Biol. Chem.* **269**, 32,721–32,724.

Tanzi R. E., Gusella J. F., Watkins P. C., Bruns G. A., St George-Hyslop P. H., Van Keuren M. L., Patterson D., Pagan S., Kurnit D. M., and Neve R. L. (1987) Amyloid β protein gene: cDNA, mRNA distribution, and genetic linkage near the Alzheimer locus. *Science* **235,** 880–884.

Tanzi R. E., St George-Hyslop P. H., and Gusella J. F. (1989) Molecular genetic approaches to Alzheimer's disease. *Trends Neurosci.* **12,** 152–158.

Wyllie A. H., Kerr J. F. R., and Currie A. R. (1980) Cell death: the significance of apoptosis. *Int. Rev. Cytol.* **68,** 251–306.

Wyllie A. H., Morris R. G., Smith A. L., and Dunlop D. (1984) Chromatin cleavage in apoptosis: association with condensed chromatin morphology and dependence on macromolecular synthesis. *J. Pathol.* **142,** 67–77.

Yankner B. A., Dawes L. R., Fisher S., Villa-Komaroff L., Oster-Granite M. L., and Neve R. L. (1989) Neurotoxicity of a fragment of the amyloid precursor associated with Alzheimer's disease. *Science* **245,** 417–420.

Detection of Cell Death in Neural Tissue and Cell Culture

*Thomas Mahalik,
Malcolm Wood, and Gregory Owens*

1. Introduction

In recent years, we have studied cell death in the developing nervous system (Owens et al., 1995), in fetal tissue grafts (Mahalik et al., 1995), and in the rodent olfactory epithelium (Mahalik, 1995). In addition, we are interested in correlating cell death in the rodent CNS with the expression of a putative death-related mRNA called RPS (Owens et al., 1991; Owens et al., 1995; Mahalik et al., 1995). In these studies we have used standard Nissl stains; fluorescent dyes, such as Hoechst 33258 which stain DNA; and the TUNEL method (Gavrieli et al., 1992), in which biotinylated deoxyUTP is incorporated into 3'-hydroxyl groups in nicked or fragmented DNA to identify apoptotic cells in tissue sections. In more recent work, we have combined the TUNEL procedure with immunocytochemistry to identify dying cells in the rodent olfactory epithelium (Mahalik, 1995). Finally, we have used modifications of the TUNEL procedure and other methods to study the aspects of cell death and apoptosis in cultures of PC12 cells and immature rodent thymocytes.

Each of the techniques mentioned above has its advantage and disadvantages. Our experience with each of these methods will be described below. In addition, the protocols for our modification of the TUNEL method is presented at the end of this chapter.

From: *Neuromethods, Vol. 29: Apoptosis Techniques and Protocols*
Ed: J. Poirier Humana Press Inc.

2. Programmed Cell Death in Neurons

Programmed cell death (PCD) is extensive in the developing nervous system. As in other tissues, neural PCD is orderly and functions to regulate cell number (Oppenheim, 1991). Cells undergoing PCD have an apoptotic morphology that is distinct from cells dying neurotically (Wyllie, 1987). Apoptosis is characterized by cell shrinkage, and by fragmentation and condensation of nuclear chromatin (Wyllie, 1987). Biochemically, DNA fragmentation is manifest as a DNA ladder on agarose gels (Cohen and Duke, 1984). At the ultrastructural level, condensed chromatin is the definitive marker for apoptosis (e.g., Chu-Wang and Oppenheim, 1978). More recently, fragmented DNA in dying cells had been visualized by using terminal transferase to add biotinylated nucleotides to free 3'-OH groups in fragmented DNA (Gavrieli et al., 1992).

The occurrence of extensive cell death has been described for several different regions in the developing CNS (*see* Oppenheim, 1991 for a review). One of the best characterized regions is the spinal cord of the chick embryo, where 40–50% of the motor neurons die between embryonic days 4 and 18 (Chu-Wang and Oppenheim, 1978; Chu-Wang and Oppenheim, 1978b; Oppenheim et al., 1978). Neuronal death in the chick spinal cord occurs after axons have reached the limb bud (Chu-Wang and Oppenheim, 1978b). Removal of the limb increases the cell death to 90% (Oppenheim et al., 1978). Conversely, the death of motor neurons is reduced, if they are supplied with an additional target with innervate (Hollyday and Hamburger, 1976). Thus, in this as in other systems, the amount of neuronal death is related to the size of the target tissue.

In the developing rat nervous system neuronal death is also common. For example, in the development striatum, 30–50% of generated neurons die during the first postnatal week (Fisher and Van der Kooy, 1991). Cell death apparently occurs in striatal neurons after they have projected to the substantia nigra (Fishell and Van der Kooy, 1991). Moreover, cell death peaks in this system on postnatal d 6 (Mahalik et al., 1994). Neuronal cell death is also prominent in the developing rodent spinal cord. In the rat thoracic spinal cord there is a massive loss of motor axons in the ventral root from E15–El9 (Harris and McCraig, 1984). Similarly, in the mouse spinal cord there is greater than 60% loss of motorneurons between E13 and birth (Lance-Jones and Landmesser, 1982). As in other systems, the bulk of the neuronal death occurs after neuronal axons their targets in the hindlimb, suggesting that the long-term cell survival depends on target-derived growth factors.

Until recently, standard histological stains, such as cresyl violet, thionin, or H&E have been used to identify apoptotic cells (e.g., *see* Chu-Wang and Oppenheim, 1978). In Nissl-stained material, chromatin is heavily stained at the periphery of a cell's nucleus. In ultrastructural studies, this staining pattern has been correlated with chromatin condensation (Chu-Wang and Oppenheim, 1978). Even with the recent introduction, histochemical methods to label fragmented DNA, electron microscopy remains the definitive method for identifying apoptotic cells. During the last several years, the TUNEL method has been used extensively in the studies of cell death in the nervous system. Our use of this method and others is described in the sections that follow.

3. Methods for Detecting Apoptotic Cells in Tissue Sections

3.1. Tissue Fixation

For all of the detection methods described below, we have used paraformaldehyde fixation and cryostat-cut frozen sections. Brains are fixed in 4% paraformaldehyde in 0.1M phosphate buffer (PB, pH 7.2–7.6). Neonatal brains are immersion-fixed in the above solution for 8–12 h at 4°C; adult animals are perfusion-fixed with 200–400 mL of the buffered paraformaldehyde solution. We prefer not to perfuse rats with buffered saline prior to the fixative. Instead, after adult rats have been deeply anesthetized, they are intracardially injected with a 1% solution of sodium nitrite, a potent vaso-dilator (Eldred et al., 1983; Mahalik et al., 1995), followed by an intracardial injection of 10,000 U of sodium heparin. The brains are removed from the cranium and typically postfixed in the 4% paraformaldehyde solution for 6–8 h at 4°C. After the fixation steps, both adult and neonatal brains are immersed in 0.1M PB containing 15% sucrose for 6– 12 h at 4°C to protect tissue from ice crystal damage.

3.2. Sectioning

The brains are blocked, and then are frozen in OCT embedding medium (Tissue Tek) on a bed of powdered dry ice. These blocks can be stored for months at –80°C prior to sectioning. The blocks are sectioned with a cryostat, and the frozen section (10–20 μm thick) are thaw-mounted on either gelatin-coated slides, or SuperFrost Plus slides (Fisher, Pittsburgh, PA). The slide-mounted tissue can be stored for months at –80°C. This method of tissue preparation is compatible with the TUNEL method, with standard histological staining methods and with immunocytochemical methods. In addition, if care is taken to eliminate RNase contamination from solutions and glassware (Blumberg, 1987), tissue sections can also be used in *in situ* hybridization experiments (e.g., *see* Owens et al., 1995).

Prior to each of the staining methods described below, slide-mounted frozen sections re brought to room temperature, and then are warmed on a slide-warmer (45–55°C) for 1 h. This ensures that the tissue sections are firmly mounted on the slides.

3. Standard Histological Stains

We have used standard histological stains, such as hematoxylin and eosin and cresyl violet to detect apoptotic cells in frozen sections of nenous tissue. The advantage of these stains is that they are easy to use and inexpensive. Established staining protocols exist for both stains (Ralis et al., 1973) and will not be detailed here. Examples of H&E-stained

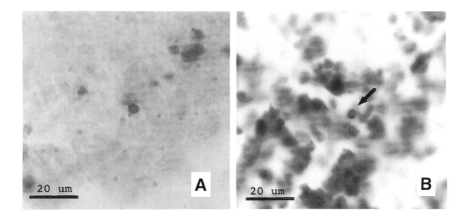

Fig. 1. Comparison of TUNEL-labeling with H&E staining. **(A)** The cerebellum of a 12-d-old weaver mutant mouse. The tissue was labeled with the modified TUNEL method described in the text. A positive cell with a doughnut morphology is highlighted by the arrow. The peroxidase-label accumulates around the periphery of the nucleus. **(B)** H&E stain of a 12-d weaver mutant. Note that the morphology of the highlighted apoptotic cell is very similar to the morphology of the TUNEL-positive cell in Fig. 1A.

apoptotic cells are presented in Fig. 1B. As shown here, the primary difference between normal cells and apoptotic cells is in the nucleus. Healthy neurons exhibit a lightly stained nucleus and a darkly stained nucleolus. In contrast, the nuclei of apoptotic cells are darkly stained; in particular, chromatin at the periphery of nuclei are stained. Staining of the cell body is very light, and in some cases absent. In more advance stages of apoptosis, darkly stained chromatin is present in the center of the nucleus, and staining of the cell body is usually absent. In our work we have correlated this staining pattern with positive labeling of fragmented DNA with biotinylated deoxyUTP (*see* Fig. 1).

4. *In Situ* Labeling of Fragmented DNA (TUNEL Method)

The study of apoptotic cell death in histological sections became a mainstay of apoptosis research when Gavrieli et al. (Gavrieli et al., 1992) introduced a method for adding biotinylated deoxyUTP to the 3'-hydroxyl end of fragmented DNA. The addition of dUTP is catalyzed by terminal deoxy transferase. The incorporated biotinylated dUTP can be detected with avidin complexed to biotin (ABC method), or with avidin tagged with rhodamine or fluorescein. We have used both methods in our work and have found that the ABC method is more sensitive when labeling cells in histological sections. For labeling cells in culture, both the ABC method and fluorescent labeling can be used with equal success. In most of our work, we have used a modified version of the TUNEL method described by Gavrieli et al. (1992). Slide mounted tissue sections are air dried and then placed in 100% methanol for 15 min. The slides are then placed in a 3% solution of hydrogen peroxide for 15 min. These two steps are critical because they quench endogenous peroxidase activity. This is particularly important in our work with neo-natal material, in which tissue is immersion-fixed; many per-oxidase-positive red blood cells are presents in this tissue, making it virtually impossible to identify apoptotic cells. In our modification of the TUNEL method, the sections are placed in $0.1M$ phosphate buffer containing 0.3% Triton X for 15 min. The slides are then rinsed for 30 min in running deionized water. Excess liquid is removed from the slides and 100 μL of terminal deoxytransferase (TdT) reaction mix-ture supplied by the manufacturer is added (Stratagene, La Jolla, CA): For each 100 μL of reaction buffer, 40 U of TdT and 2 nmol of biotinylated deoxyUTP are used. The sections are incubated for 90 min at 37°C. The slides are washed for 30 min in PBS, and then incubated in avidin complexed to biotin (1:200) in PBS for at least 2 h at room temperature. After another wash step, the slides are reacted for 10 min in 3,3'-diaminobensidine (Sigma, St. Louis, MO, 25 mg/50 mL) and 0.0075% hydrogen peroxide. The sections are washed in PBS, rinsed in deionized water, and air dried. The slides are then dehydrated in increasing concentrations of ethanol, defatted in Americlear (a xylene substitute, Stephen Scien-tific, Riverdale, NJ), and coverslipped with DPX mounting medium. As a control, the tissue is reacted in the steps described above, except that terminal deoxytransferase is left out of the reaction step.

Examples of TUNEL-labeled cells in the cerebellum of a 12-d-old *weaver* mutant mouse are shown in Fig. 1A. In *weaver* neonates, granule cells fail to migrate to the granule cell layer; instead they move to the edge of the external granule layer where they undergo apoptotic cell death. Recent work by Grassl et al. (1995) suggests that the TUNEL procedure can label necrotic cells under some conditions. Therefore, it is critical that the morphology of TUNEL-positive cells is taken into account before identifying the cell as apoptotic. By comparing Figs. 1A and 1B, it can be seen that the morphology of the TUNEL-positive cell (Fig. 1A, arrow) is quite similar to the H&E-stained apoptotic cell in Fig. 1B (arrow). The best morphological marker of apoptosis in TUNEL-labeled material is the accumulation of peroxidase reaction product around the periphery of a cell's nucleus (Fig. 2, cells A and C). In more advanced stages of apoptosis, small, TUNEL-positive globules may be present in the center of a cell (Fig. 2, cell B).

4.1. Fluorescent TUNEL-Labeling of Cultured Cells

We have also used the TUNEL method to label apoptotic cells in cultures of immature thymocytes and PC12 cells. Immature thymocytes are obtained from 3–4-wk-old Sprague-Dawley rats (Harlan Laboratories, Zeist, The Netherlands). The thymus is removed and the cells are dissociated by pushing the thymus through a fine mesh nylon screen. The thymocytes are then plated at a density of 1×10^7 cells/mL in RPMI 1640 medium containing 10% fetal bovine serum with L-glutamine and $NaHCO_3$. To induce death, 1 μM dexamethasone was added to the cultures for 10 h. The cells were fixed for 60 min in 4% panaformaldehyde on $0.1M$ phosphate buffer. The cells were washed thoroughly in distilled water and reacted as described above for tissue sections. In our cell culture experiments, aliquots of cells are place in 300 μL Eppendorf tubes. After each step in the labeling procedure, the cells are spun down with a microcentrifuge, and the liq-

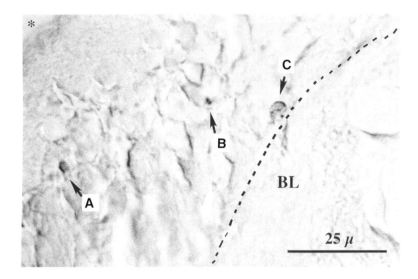

Fig. 2. Reflective confocal imaging of TUNEL-positive cells in the rat olfactory epithelium. Two cells (A and C) exhibit accumulation of reaction product at the periphery of nuclei resulting in a doughnut morphology typical of apoptotic cells. Cell B in which labeling consists of two small globules, may be in a more advance stage of apoptosis. An advantage of bright-field confocal imaging is that unlabeled cells are clearly visible. BL = Basal Lamina. The surface (*) of the epithelium is to the top left of the figure.

uid is aspirated. To detect incorporated biotinylated dUTP, the cells are incubated with fluorescein-conjugated avidin in PBS (diluted 1:100, Jackson Laboratories, Bar Harbor, ME) for 2 h at room temperature. After three wash steps, a 10–15-μL aliquot of cells can be placed on a microscope slide and coverslipped with a glycerol-phosphate buffer moisture (1 part 0.1M phosphate buffer, 9 parts glycerol). All cells can be visualized with a rhodamine filter set if they are labeled with a dilute solution of cresyl violet; apoptotic cells are visualized with a fluorescein filter set. In our work we add 0.5 μL of a stock cresyl violet solution to a 30-μL suspension of cells. The cells are then washed and placed on slides. Figure 3A shows cresyl violet-stained thymocytes illuminated with a rhodamine filter set.

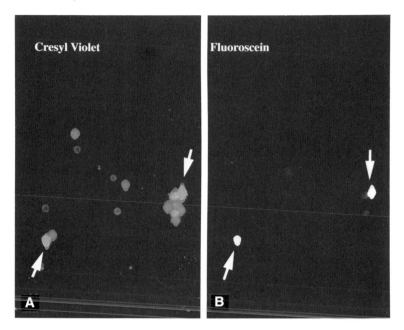

Fig. 3. TUNEL-labeling of immature thymocytes in cell cultures. **(A)** Thymocytes were stained with a dilute solution of cresyl violet that labels all cells. Arrows highlight double-labeled cells. The cells are visualized with the rhodamine filter cube. **(B)** Fluorescent TUNEL-labeling of cells visualized with fluorescein-tagged avidin. Two apoptotic cells are highlighted by arrows.

Figure 3B (arrow) shows two TUNEL-positive cells labeled with fluorescein-tagged avidin. This double labeling should be adaptable to fluorescent automated cell sorting (FACS).

4.2. Combined TUNEL Labeling and Immunocytochemistry

We have examined cell death in the olfactory epithelium of the rat. In the rodent epithelium, neurons are generated and undergo cell death throughout the lifespan of the organism (Graziadei and Graziadei, 1979; Farbman, 1990). One goal of our work was to identify those olfactory cells that underwent apoptotic cell death. To do this, we combined the TUNEL-labeling method described above with immunocytochemistry for three different markers of olfactory neuron development: keratin, GAP43, and olfactory marker protein (OMP). The keratin antibody labels only the basal cells of the epithelium (Moll, 1982); the GAP43 antibody labels differentiated, immature neurons (Verhaagen et al., 1989), and the olfactory marker protein antibody labels mature receptor neurons.

Slide-mounted frozen sections of olfactory epithelium are TUNEL-labeled as described above. The sections are then washed thoroughly in PBS, incubated in PBS containing 2% normal serum (species depends on the species in which the 2° antiserum is made), and then placed in the 1° antiserum for 16–48 h. After 3–4 wash steps in PBS, the slides are exposed to a fluorescently tagged 2° antiserum. We typically use antisera from Jackson Laboratories, diluted 1:200 to 1:1000 in PBS containing 2% of the appropriate normal serum. For the wash steps, the slides are placed in koplin jars. For the antibody incubation steps, the slides are placed in plexiglass chambers with moist filter paper. We typically use 100–200 µL of antibody solution per tissue section.

The cells of the olfactory epithelium are densely packed in a psuedostratified epithelium. In our double labeling work, the cytoarchitecture of the epithelium made it difficult to resolve individual double-labeled cells with conventional bright-field and fluorescent microscopy. Therefore, we used simultaneous reflective and fluorescent confocal imaging on a Bio-Rad (Richmond, CA), MRC600 scanning confocal microscope. As Figs. 2 and 4 show, we were able to obtain high-quality, bright-field images of peroxidase-labeled apoptotic cells. With reflective confocal imaging, it is possible to optically section through a peroxidase-labeled nucleus to determine the determine the distribution of label nucleus to determine the distribution of label within cells. This enabled us to show that TUNEL-positive cells in the epithelium had apoptotic morphology. In the confocal image shown in Fig. 2, the reaction product is most intense at the peripheries of cells A and C; in cell B, which may be in a more advanced stage apoptosis, the reaction product is present in two small globules at the center of a cell ghost. Another

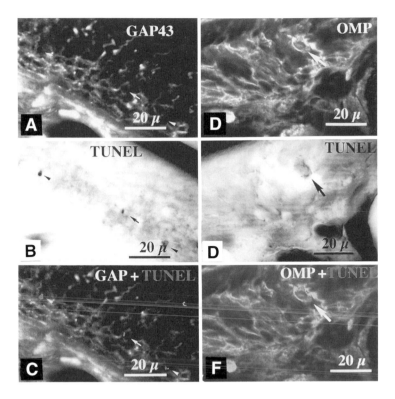

Fig. 4. Reflective and fluorescent confocal microscopy of TUNEL and immunocytochemically labeled cells in the rat olfactory epithelium. **(A)** A cluster of positive cells, one of which (arrow) is TUNEL-positive. The arrowheads show the location of TUNEL-positive cells that are GAP43 negative. **(B)** A bright-field, confocal image of TUNEL-labeling. **(C)** A composite image illustrating the relationship between TUNEL (red patches) and GAP43 labeling. **(D)** An OMP neuron (arrow) that is also TUNEL-positive. **(E)** Bright-field image of TUNEL-labeling. **(F)** A composite image showing the relationship between TUNEL-labeling (RED) and OMP immunoreactivity.

advantage of reflective confocal imaging is that some morphological details of unlabeled cells (Fig. 2, cell D) are visible.

Confocal microscopy is also invaluable when TUNEL-labeling is combined with immunocytochemistry. One advantage is that it is possible to correctly align dark-field and bright-field images, making it much easier to identify double-labeled cells. Figure 4 shows an example of a double labeling experiment in which olfactory epithelium was labeled with OMP or GAP43 antibodies after apoptotic cells were labeled with the TUNEL procedure. The arrows in Fig. 4A, C highlight GAP43 and OMP-positive cells respectively. Bright-field images of the same sections show TUNEL reaction product (Fig. 4B, 4E, arrows) in the nuclei of these two cells. The double labeling is better illustrated in Fig. 4C, E, in which regions of TUNEL-labeling from the bright-field images were thresholded and added to the dark-field image (Fig. 4B,C, gray shading).

5. TUNEL Procedure: Detailed Protocols

5.1. Procedures

1. Slide-mounted cryostat sections (10–20 µm thick) are placed on a slide warmer at 45°C for 60 min.
2. Place slides in 100% methanol for 15 min.
3. Place slides in 3% hydrogen peroxide for 15 min.
4. Incubate slides in 0.3% Triton-X 100 in phosphate-buffered aline (PBS) for 15 min.
5. Rinse thoroughly in running deionized water.
6. Terminal transferase addition of biotinylated dUTP to fragmented DNA (100 µL reaction).
    a. 20 µL 5X terminal transferase reaction buffer (Stratagene).
    b. 2 µL (40 U) terminal deoxytransferase (Strategene, Mannheim, Germany).
    c. 2 µL (2 nmol) biotinylated deoxyUTP (Boehringer).
    d. 76 µL sterile distilled water.
    e. Incubate at 37°C for 1.5–2 h.
7. Rinse in PBS 3 × 10 min.
8. Incubate in avidin biotinylated peroxidase complex (Vectastain, 1:100 dilution) for 2 h at room temperature.
9. Rinse in PBS.
10. DAB reaction: 25 mg 3,3'-diaminobensidine (Sigma) per 50 mL PBS, with 25 µL 3.0% hydrogen peroxide for 10 min.
11. Rinse in deionized water, dehydrate, defat, and coverslip.

5.2. For Combined TUNEL and Immunocytochemical Labeling

1. After DAB step, wash in PBS 3 × 10 min.
2. Block in PBS containing 2% normal serum for 30 min to 1 h (e.g., rabbit, mouse or donkey, depends on the species in which the 2° antiserum was made).
3. Incubate in the primary antiserum for 24–48 h in the above buffer. We use 100–200 µL of the primary antibody solution per slides. The slides are placed in humid chambers and incubated at 4°C.
4. Wash slides in PBS 3 × 10 min.
5. Incubate in appropriate fluorescent 2° antibody for 1–2 h at room temperature.
6. Wash in PBS 3 × 10 min.
7. Coverslip with glycerol phosphate buffer mixture.

Acknowledgments

This work was supported by an NIH Shannon Award to Thomas Mahalik.

References

Blumberg D. D. (1987) Creating a ribonuclease-free environment. *Methods Enzymol.* **153,** 20–24.

Chu-Wang I.-W. and Oppenheim R. W. (1978) Cell death of motorneurons in the chick embryo spinal cord I. A light and electron microscopic study of naturally occurring and induced cell loss during development. *J. Comp Neurol.* **177,** 33–59.

Chu-Wang I.-W. and Oppenheim R. W. (1978) Cell death of motorneurons in the chick embryo spinal cord II. A quantitative and qualitative analysis of degeneration in the ventral dorsal root, including evidence for axon outgrowth and limb innervation prior to cell death. *J. Comp. Neurol.* **177,** 59–86.

Eldred W. D., Zucker C., Karten H., and Yazulla S. J. (1983) Comparison of fixation and penetration enhancement techniques for use in ultrastructural immunocytochemistry. *J. Histochem. Cytochem.* **31,** 258–292.

Farbman A. I. (1990) Olfactory neurogenesis: genetic or environmental controls. *TINS* **13,** 362–365.

Fishell G. and Van der Kooy D. (1991) Pattern formation in the striatum: neurons with early projections to the substantia nigra survive the cell death period. *J. Comp Neurol.* **312,** 33–42.

Graziadei P. P. C. and Graziadei M. (1979) Neurogenesis and neuron regeneration in the olfactory system of animals. I. morphological aspects of differentiation and structural organization of the olfactory sensory neurons. *J. Neurocytol.* **8,** 1–18.

Harris A. J. and McCraig C. D. (1984) Motorneuron death and motor unit size during embryonic development of the rat. *J. Neurosci.* **4,** 13–24.

Hollyday M. and Hamburger V. (1976) Reduction of naturally occurring motorneuron loss by enlargement of the periphery. *J. Comp. Neurol.* **170,** 311–320.

Lance-Jones C. and Landmesser L. (1982) Motorneuron cell death in the developing lumbar spinal cord of the mouse. *Dev. Brain Res.* **4,** 473–479.

Mahalik T. J., Hahn W. E., Clayton G. H., and Owens G. P. (1994) Programmed cell death in the striatum of the neonatal rat. *Soc. Neurosci. Abs.* **20,** 688.

Mahalik T. J. (1995) Basal cells, immature and mature neurons undergo programmed cell death in the rat olfactory epithelium. *Soc. Neurosci. Abs.* **21,** 2019.

Mahalik T. J., Hahn W. E., Clayton G. H., and Owens G. P. (1995) The expression of thymocyte death-related mRNA is associated with cell death in developing grafts of fetal substantia nigra. *Exp. Neurol.* **129,** 27–36.

Moll R., Franke W. W., Schiller D. L., Geiger B., and Kepler R. (1982) The catalog of human cytokeratins: patterns of expression in normal epithelia, tumors and cultured cells. *Cell* **31,** 11–24.

Owens G. P., Mahalik T. J., and Hahn W. E. (1995) Expression of the death-associated gene RP8 in granule neurons undergoing postnatal cell death in the cerebellum of weaver mice. *Dev. Brain Res.* **86,** 35–47.

Owens G. P., Hahn W. E., and Cohen J. J. (1991) Identification of mRNAs associated with programmed cell death in immature thymocytes. *Mol. Cell Biol.* **11,** 4177–4188.

Oppenheim R. W. (1991) Cell death during development of the nervous system. *Ann. Rev. Neraosci.* **14,** 453–501.

Oppenheim R. W., Chu-Wang I.-W., and Maderdrut J. L. (1978) Cell death of motorneurons in the chick embryo spinal cord iii, the differentiation of motorneurons prior to their induced degeneration following limb-bud removal. *J. Comp. Neurol.* **177,** 87–112.

Verhaagen J., Oestreicher A. B., and Margolis F. L. (1989) The expression of the growth associated protein B50/GAP43 in the olfactory system of neonatal and adult rats. *J. Neurosci.* **9,** 683–691.

Wyllie A. H. (1987) Cell death in tissue regulation. *Pathology* **153,** 313–316.

Cultured Cerebellar Granule Neurons as a Model of Neuronal Apoptosis

Guang-Mei Yan and Steven M. Paul

1. Introduction

Apoptosis is one type of programmed cell death responsible for the physiological elimination of various cell populations during development (Wyllie, 1988). It has been estimated that up to 50% or more of vertebrate neurons in the central nervous system (CNS) die during embryonic development and/or early postnatal maturation via programmed cell death (Raff et al., 1993). There is increasing evidence that apoptosis may also be triggered pathologically in the adult CNS and may mediate the nonphysiological death of neurons characteristic of various neurodegenerative disorders, such as Alzheimer's disease (Barinaga, 1993), and that which occurs following ischemic, traumatic, or chemical injury of the CNS (Yoshitatsu et al., 1994; Yan et al., 1995a).

Cerebellar granule neurons, the principle interneurons of the cerebellum, are among the most abundant neuronal phenotype in the mammalian CNS (Ito, 1984a). These neurons contain glutamate as their primary neurotransmitter and express both N-methyl-D-aspartate (NMDA) and non-NMDA glutamate receptors on their dendrites and perikarya (Garthwaite et al., 1986; Burgoyne and Cambray-Deakin, 1988). During cerebellar development, granule neurons are generated postnatally in the external germinal layer where they differentiate, migrate in approx 3 d to the granule neuron layer and are finally innervated by mossy fiber axons

From: *Neuromethods, Vol. 29: Apoptosis Techniques and Protocols*
Ed: J. Poirier Humana Press Inc.

(Altman, 1972). There is evidence that mossy fiber axons from the dorsal pontine nuclei of the brainstem, which innervate cerebellar granule neurons, utilize acetylcholine as a primary neurotransmitter (Ito, 1984a,b). Granule neurons in turn innervate Purkinje cell dendrites via their long, parallel fiber axons (Ito, 1984a). There is a rather precise stoichiometry between the number of Purkinje cells and granule neurons in the adult cerebellum (Ito, 1984a). Postmitotic granule neurons can be readily maintained in vitro in their fully differentiated state for several weeks if depolarized with high concentrations of K^+ (25 mM) (Gallo et al., 1987) or by exposure to the excitatory amino acids, glutamate, or NMDA (Balázs et al., 1988).

If, on the other hand, cultured cerebellar granule neurons are exposed to nondepolarizing culture conditions shortly after plating they will die over the ensuing 2–3 d. The death of cultured cerebellar granule neurons under such conditions occurs via apoptosis (Yan et al., 1994; D'Mello et al., 1993). Given the relative homogeneity of these cultures, and the ease at which apoptosis can be reliably induced, cultured cerebellar granule neurons have proven to be a fascile in vitro model system for studying neuronal apoptosis.

2. Preparation of Cultured Rat Cerebellar Granule Neurons and Assessment of Neuronal Viability

Cerebellar granule neurons can be prepared from 8-d-old Sprague-Dawley rat pups (16–19 g) as previously described (Yan et al., 1994). Briefly, cells are dissociated from freshly dissected cerebella by mechanical disruption in the presence of trypsin and DNase and then plated in poly-L-lysine (5 µg/mL)-coated 35-mm culture plates (Costar, Cambridge, MA). Cells are seeded at a density of 1.5–1.8 × 10⁶ cells/mL (2 mL/dish) in basal modified Eagle's medium containing 10% fetal bovine serum (heat inactivated), 0.1 µg/mL gentamicin, 2 mM L-glutamine, and 25 mM KCl. Cytosine arabinoside 10 µM (Ara-C, 200X solution prepared with the plating medium) is added to the culture medium after 24 h to arrest the growth of nonneuronal cells. D-Glucose (100 µL of

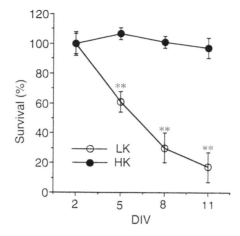

Fig. 1. The effects of LK (5 mM) vs HK (25 mM) culture medium on granule neuron survival in vitro. Neurons from PND8 dissociated rat cerebelli were cultured in 35-mm dishes and cultured in either LK or HK medium. Neuronal viability was assessed by fluorescein diacetate vital staining and visual counting of viable neurons as described by Yan et al., 1994 and the text. Data represent the mean ± SEM of triplicate cultures from two separate experiments (**$p < 0.001$, ANOVA followed by Bonferroni/Dunn) and are from Yan et al. (1994) taken with permission.

a 100 mM solution prepared in sterile water) is added to the cultures on d 7 and every fourth day thereafter.

Viable granule neurons are quantified after staining with fluorescein formed from fluorescein diacetate, which is deesterified only by living cells (*see* Yan et al., 1994 and references therein for details). Briefly, after incubation with 10 µg/mL of fluorescein diacetate (Sigma, St. Louis, MO; a 1000X stock solution is made in acetone and the working solution is made by dilution [1:1000] with phosphate-buffered saline [PBS, pH 7.2]), neurons are examined and photographed under UV light microscopy and the number of neurons/representative low-power field (10× magnification) are counted from the photomicrographs. Values are generally expressed as the percent control (vehicle treated) cultures in each experiment.

As can be seen in Fig. 1, rat cerebellar granule neurons are effectively maintained in vitro when harvested at postnatal d 8 (PND8) and cultured in high concentrations of K^+ (25 mM) (HK) (Gallo et al., 1987). By contrast, when cerebellar granule neurons are cultured in physiological K^+ (5 mM) (LK), they die over the ensuing 3–11 d (Yan et al., 1994).

It has been previously demonstrated that addition of fresh serum-containing medium to established cultures of cerebellar granule neurons results in a delayed type of neurotoxicity, which is blocked by NMDA receptor antagonists (Schramm et al., 1990). This neurotoxicity does not occur if conditioned "sister culture medium" is used (Yan et al., 1994). Figure 2 shows the effect of replacing HK medium with fresh LK or HK medium to established granule neuron cultures. Replacement with either HK or LK medium results in substantial neuronal death (50–80%) within 48–72 h. The addition of the noncompetitive NMDA receptor antagonist (+)5-methyl-10,11-dihydro-5H-dibenzo[a,d]cyclohepten-5,10-imine maleate (MK-801) however, completely prevents neuronal death induced by fresh HK medium exchange (Fig. 2). Thus, medium exchange to fresh HK medium results in excitotoxic neuronal death which is blocked by NMDA receptor antagonists. When HK medium is replaced with conditioned LK (cLK) medium, the same magnitude and time-course of cell death as with fresh LK medium is observed (Fig. 2). However, whereas the neurotoxic effect(s) of changing to cLK medium is completely blocked by increasing the concentration of KCl to 25 mM, MK-801 fails to affect cell death induced by cLK medium exchange (Fig. 2). These data confirm that a reduced K^+ concentration *per se,* and not some unknown factor present in LK medium, is responsible for neuronal death.

3. Biochemical Evidence for Neuronal Apoptosis of Cultured Rat Cerebellar Granule Neurons

For these experiments, granule neurons (3×10^7) are cultured in 100×10-mm dishes and collected in cold, phosphate-buffered saline (PBS, pH 7.2). After removing the medium and washing once with cold PBS, the cells are centrifuged at

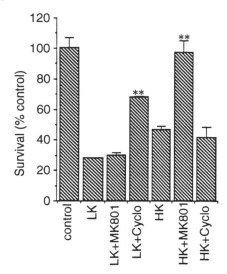

Fig. 2. Effects of cycloheximide, actinomycin D, and MK-801 on neurotoxicity induced by changing medium to fresh LK or HK medium. Neurons from PND8 dissociated rat cerebelli were cultured in 35-mm dishes for 7 d as described in the text. Cycloheximide (1.0 µg/mL), actinomycin D (0.05 µg/mL), and/or MK-801 (1 µM) were added to fresh medium either containing 5 mM K$^+$ or 25 mM K$^+$. After 48 h, neuronal viability was assessed by fluorescein diacetate staining and visual counting of viable neurons. Note switching to either fresh LK or HK medium induces prominent neurotoxicity. LK medium toxicity was attenuated by cycloheximide (**$p < 0.001$), but was unaffected by MK-801. In contrast, HK medium toxicity was blocked by MK-801 (**$p < 0.001$), but not by cycloheximide and/or actinomycin D (not shown). Data are from Yan et al. (1994) taken with permission.

5000g for 5 min and the pellet lysed in 600 µL of a buffer consisting of 10 mM Tris-HCl, 10 mM EDTA, and 0.2% Triton X-100, pH 7.5. After 15 min on ice, the lysate is centrifuged at 12,000g for 10 min at 4°C. The supernatant (containing RNA and fragmented DNA, but not intact chromatin) is extracted first with phenol and then with phenol-chloroform:isoamyl alcohol (24:1). Sodium acetate is added to the aqueous phase to a final concentration of 300 mM and nucleic acids are precipitated with 1 vol of isopropanol overnight. The pellet is rinsed with 70% ethanol, air dried, and dissolved

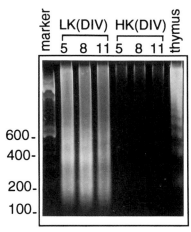

Fig. 3. DNA gel electrophoresis shows internucleosomal DNA fragmentation of cerebellar granule neurons cultured in HK medium and switched to LK, but not to HK medium. Data are from Yan et al. (1994) and are taken with permission.

in 15 µL of 10 mM Tris-HCl/1 mM EDTA, pH 7.5. After adding RNase A (0.6 mg/mL, at 37°C for 30 min), the sample is electrophoresed in a 2% agarose gel with TBE buffer. DNA can be visualized with ethidium bromide staining. As a positive control, freshly isolated thymocytes are obtained from 4-wk-old rats, separated using wire mesh, and collected in BME with 10% fetal bovine serum. Thymocytes are then incubated with dexamethasone (1.0 µM) at 37°C for 3 h. The cells are collected, washed once with PBS containing 5 mM MgCl$_2$, and resuspended in Tris/EDTA buffer to a final concentration of 5 × 10^7 cells/mL. Subsequent lysing and DNA extraction procedures are identical to those described above for cerebellar granule neurons.

Figure 3 shows that agarose gel electrophoresis of DNA extracted from granule neurons maintained in either HK or LK medium reveals the characteristic fragmentation pattern of nucleosomal-size DNA in cells maintained in LK but not HK conditions (Fig. 3) (Wyllie et al., 1980, 1981, 1988). This same pattern of fragmentation is observed with DNA obtained from rat thymocytes following incubation with dexamethasone (1 μM for 3 h; Fig. 3). Little DNA fragmentation is observed in DNA prepared from HK neurons (Fig. 3), although we occasionally observe some internucleosomal fragmentation of DNA prepared from cultures established from older pups (>PND 10).

4. Morphological Evidence for Neuronal Apoptosis in Cultured Rat Cerebellar Granule Neurons

Morphological criteria have been extensively used to distinguish necrotic vs apoptotic death of many cell types. Morphological changes that define apoptosis include cell shrinkage, cytoplasmic blebbing, heterochromatic clumping, and condensation of nuclear chromatin or aggregation at the nuclear membrane (Wylli, 1988; Wyllie et al., 1981). The most common methods currently used to detect such changes are microscopic visualization using Nomarski optics, fluorescent staining of nuclear chromatin using Hoechst 33258 (or other fluorescent dyes), and *in situ* labeling of the 3'-OH end of the fragmented DNA, which is characteristic of apoptotic cells (Yan et al., 1994, 1995c,d).

For visualization using Nomarski optics, cerebellar granule neurons are cultured on 20-mm glass coverslips using the same protocol as described above (Yan et al., 1994). As can be seen in Fig. 5, cerebellar granule neurons maintained in LK medium for 5–11 d in vitro (DIV) display morphological features characteristic of apoptotic cells, including cytoplasmic blebbing and heterochromatic clumping (Fig. 5A,B). Sixteen hours after switching from HK to cLK medium the neurons also show typical apoptotic morphology (Fig. 5D) and the apoptosis induced by cLK can be completely blocked by increasing the final concentration of KCl to 25 mM (Fig. 5C).

For staining of nuclear chromatin, cerebellar granule neurons are cultured in 35-mm tissue culture dishes as described above (*see* Yan et al., 1994). After removing the medium, the neurons are rinsed once with cold PBS (pH 7.2) and fixed for 10 min with 4% formaldehyde in PBS at 4°C, washed with distilled water, and dried at room temperature.

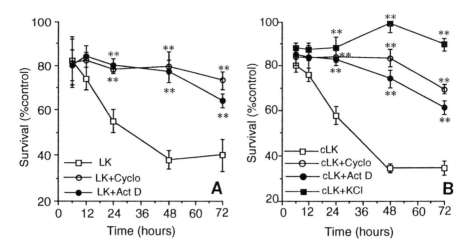

Fig. 4. Time course of apoptotic death induced in cerebellar granular neurons by switching to LK medium and the enhancement of granule neuron survival by inhibitors of RNA and protein synthesis. **(A)** Granule neuron death induced by switching HK cells at 8 DIV to fresh LK medium for 6–72 h in the presence or absence of either cycloheximide (1.0 μg/mL) or actinomycin D (0.05 μg/mL). Values represent the mean ± SEM of percent control (conditioned HK) from triplicate cultures at each time point from two separate experiments. Both cycloheximide and actinomycin D significantly attenuate (**$p < 0.001$ by ANOVA, Bonferroni/Dunn) granule neuron death induced by LK medium exchange. **(B)** Cycloheximide (1.0 μg/mL), actinomycin D (0.05 μg/mL) and KCl (20 mM), block (**$p < 0.001$ by ANOVA, Bonferroni/Dunn) granule neuron death induced by conditioned LK (cLK) medium. Values represent the mean ± SEM of percent control (conditioned HK) from triplicate cultures at each time point from two separate experiments. Note approx 70% cell loss in cLK medium at 48–72 h compared to approx 10–30% with KCl, cycloheximide and actinomycin D, respectively. Data are from Yan et al. (1994) and are taken with permission.

Cells can be readily stained with Hoechst 33258 (5 μg/mL) for 5 min, washed, and dried (Yan et al., 1994). Photomicrographs are randomly obtained and can be quantified if necessary by a blind observer using (in our laboratory) a Zeiss Axiophot microscope. Figure 5F shows the characteristic condensation of nuclear chromatin (and aggregation at the nuclear membrane) observed in cultured cerebellar granule neurons undergoing apoptosis after staining with the fluorescent dye Hoechst 33258.

For *in situ* labeling of the 3'-OH end of fragmented DNA which is characteristic of apoptotic neurons, cerebellar granule neurons are cultured on poly-L-lysine-coated 13 mm coverslips using the same protocol as described above. At 8 DIV, neurons are switched to cLK medium, with or without various drugs as indicated (generally for 24 h). After removing the medium, the neurons are rinsed once with cold PBS (pH 7.2) and fixed for 10 min with 4% formaldehyde in PBS at room temperature, washed with distilled water, and dried at room temperature. The coverslips are fixed onto glass slides and dehydrated to 70% ethanol at 4°C. Labeling of the 3'-OH end of fragmented DNA is carried out according to the protocol provided by the supplier (Oncor, Gaithersburg, MD). Briefly, the fixed neurons, after quenching in 2.0% H_2O_2 in PBS and then equilibrated with 1X of the supplied equilibration buffer, are incubated with 54 µL of working strength TdT enzyme solution directly on the specimen in a humidified chamber at 37°C for 60 min. The reaction is stopped by the supplied stop/wash buffer at 37°C for 30 min and the specimen washed three times with PBS. Antidigoxigenin-peroxidase solution is layered on each coverslip and incubated at room temperature for 30 min. Color development is carried out using a H_2O_2/DAB solution and methyl green is used to counterstain the neurons. Photomicrographs can be randomly obtained by a blind observer using (in our laboratory) a Zeiss Axiophot microscope (Fig. 6 and Wyllie, 1980).

5. Inhibitors of Macromolecular Synthesis Block Apoptosis of Cultured Cerebellar Granule Neurons

In many cells, apoptosis is an active process that requires *de novo* RNA and protein synthesis and is, therefore, blocked (or delayed) by inhibitors of RNA and/or protein synthesis (Wyllie, 1988; Cohen and Duke, 1984). As can be seen in Figs. 2 and 4, both cycloheximide and actinomycin D greatly attenu-

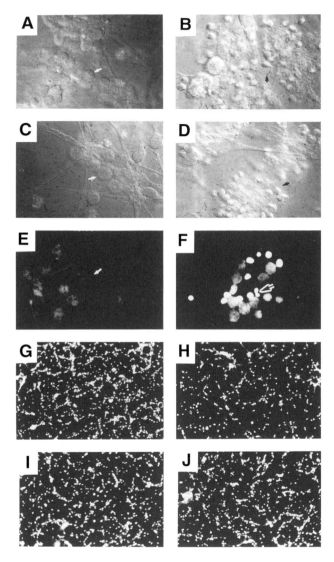

Fig. 5. **(A–D)** Apoptosis of cerebellar granule neurons cultured in nondepolarizing (LK) conditions revealed by Nomarski optics. Cerebellar granule neurons were prepared as described in text and exposed to HK (A) or LK (B) conditions for 8 DIV. HK neurons (B) show normal granule cell morphology. The LK neurons (B) show typical morphology of apoptotic cells including cell shrinkage, cytoplasmic blebbing, changes in nuclear refractivity, and reduction in neural network. In (C) and (D), HK cultures were switched to conditioned LK (cLK) medium supplemented with 20 m*M* KCl (C) or cLK medium alone (D).

ate neuronal death induced by switching HK neurons to either fresh (Figs. 2 and 4A) or conditioned LK medium (Fig. 4B).

6. Fast and Slow Neurotransmitters Regulate Apoptosis of Cerebellar Neurons

Cerebellar granule neurons can be maintained in primary culture in LK medium by adding subtoxic concentrations of glutamate or NMDA (Balázs et al., 1988). Exposure of granule neurons to these excitatory amino acids results in long-lasting membrane depolarization and elevations in $[Ca^{2+}]_i$ (Courtney et al., 1990; Koike et al., 1989). If granule neurons (PND 8) are cultured in LK medium, the addition of glutamate (15 μM) or NMDA (150 μM) greatly enhances survival over the ensuing 8 d. The addition of MK-801 (1 μM) (along with NMDA or glutamate), however, results in a marked increase in cell death (Yan et al., 1994). The latter is again markedly attenuated by coincubation with cycloheximide and is associated with the DNA fragmentation pattern characteristic of apoptosis (Yan et al., 1994). MK-801 alone fails to induce apoptosis in neurons maintained in HK conditions. However, the addition of MK-801 to LK neurons either alone, or in combination with glutamate or NMDA, results in even greater neuronal death compared to LK medium alone. The latter

---

Fig. 5. *(continued from previous page)* Again note apoptotic morphology in neurons in (D) but not (C). White arrows indicate neurons with normal morphology, whereas black arrows indicate apoptotic neurons. In **(E)** and **(F)**, HK and LK neurons respectively were stained with the fluorescent dye Hoechst 33258 to detect the typical fragmented nucleus and condensed nuclear chromatin of apoptotic neurons. Stained neurons were visualized under UV illumination (1000×). Normal (white arrows) and apoptotic nuclei (black arrows) are indicated. **(G–J)** Fluorescein diacetate staining of cerebellar granule neurons cultured in HK conditions for 8 DIV (G) were then switched to cLK medium supplemented with 20 mM KCl, (H) cLK medium alone, (I) cLK medium plus cycloheximide (1 μg/mL) and (J) cLK media plus actinomycin D (0.05 μg/mL). Note the marked loss of neurons in cLK media (compared to cLK + KCl) and the protective effects of both cycloheximide and actinomycin D.

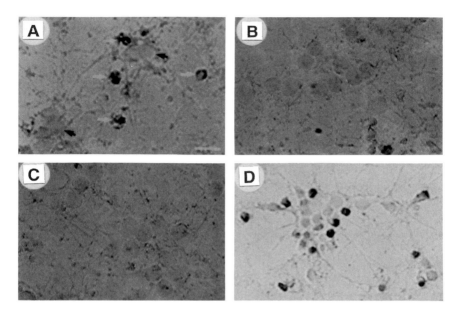

Fig. 6. *In situ* labeling of apoptotic neurons. Cerebellar granule neurons were cultured on poly-L-lysine-coated 13-mm coverslips as described in text. At 8 DIV, the neurons were switched to cLK medium with or without various drugs at the concentrations indicated for 16 h: **(A)** cLK alone; **(B)** cLK+K⁺; **(C)** cLK+CTX (2.0 µg/mL); **(D)** cLK+mastoparan (15 µM). Note the positively staining neurons (dark brown; white arrows) and the normal neurons with only weak green counter-staining (black arrows). Bar = 25 µm.

suggests that endogenous glutamate released from LK neurons may attenuate the neurotoxicity induced by nondepolarizing conditions. The nonNMDA glutamate receptor antagonist 6-cyano-7-nitroquinoxaline-2,3-dione (CNQX) also antagonizes the actions of glutamate in preventing cell death in LK medium, resulting in internucleosomal DNA fragmentation (Yan et al., 1994). Finally, incubation of LK neurons with kainate (50 µM) also increases neuronal survival and the latter is blocked by CNQX (20 µM) (Yan et al., 1994). Thus, activation of either NMDA or nonNMDA glutamate receptors can block apoptosis of cerebellar granule neurons.

In both rodents and humans it appears that mossy fiber axons from the dorsal pontine nuclei of the brainstem, which innervate cerebellar granule neurons, utilize acetylcholine (Ach) as a primary neurotransmitter (Ito, 1984a,b). In addition, cerebellar granule neurons express both nicotinic (nAchR) (Pabreza et al., 1991) and muscarinic-cholinergic receptors (mAchR), mainly the m2 and m3 subtypes (Aloso et al., 1990; Fukamauchi et al., 1993). Given our recent findings that subtoxic concentrations of the fast neurotransmitters glutamate and N-methyl-D-aspartate (NMDA), acting at ionotropic glutamate receptors, prevent apoptosis of cultured cerebellar granule neurons (Yan et al., 1994), we investigated whether Ach itself would affect the survival of cultured cerebellar granule neurons. Exposure of cultured cerebellar granule neurons maintained under nondepolarizing conditions to the muscarinic-cholinergic receptor (mAchR) agonists, carbachol and muscarine, results in a concentration- and time-dependent inhibition of apoptosis (Yan et al., 1995d). The nAchR agonist (-) nicotine fails to mimic, and the nAchR antagonist dihydro-β-erythroidine fails to antagonize, the survival-promoting effects of carbachol. By contrast, relatively low concentrations of atropine completely prevent the effects of carbachol in blocking apoptotic death of cultured granule neurons (Yan et al., 1995d). Moreover, the m1 and m2 preferring mAchR antagonists, pirenzepine and gallamine fail to reverse the effects of carbachol, the m3 preferring antagonist, 4-DAMP, completely blocks the survival-promoting effects of carbachol (Yan et al., 1995d). These data demonstrate that activation of the mAchR (most likely of the m3 subtype) blocks apoptosis of cultured cerebellar granule neurons. The antiapoptotic effects of mAchR agonists are not indirectly mediated via glutamate release from granule neurons since antagonists of either NMDA or non-NMDA glutamate receptors, fail to affect the anti-apoptotic effects of carbachol or muscarine (Yan et al., 1995d). Moreover, exposure of cultured cerebellar granule neurons to anti-apoptotic concentrations of carbachol, in contrast to high concentrations of K^+ or glutamate receptor agonists, results in only a small and transient elevation in intracellular Ca^{2+} as measured by fura-2 microfluorimetry (Yan et al., 1995d). A recent study by Nicoletti and colleagues has also shown that metabotropic glutamate receptor agonists (as well as muscariniccholinergic receptor agonists) block apoptosis of cerebellar granule neurons (Copani et al., 1995). Further, Lindenboim et al. recently reported that activation of muscarinic-cholinergic receptors inhibits apoptosis in neuronal PC12N1 cells which stably express cloned m1 mAchR (Lindenboim et al., 1995). Thus, slow neurotransmitters, such as Ach acting via their cognate G-protein coupled receptors may prevent neuronal apoptosis in the developing (and perhaps adult) CNS.

In addition to depolarizing conditions or fast or slow neurotransmitters D'Mello and colleagues (1993) have recently found that growth factors regulate apoptosis of cultured cerebellar granule neurons. These investigators have reported that insulin-like growth factor I (IGF-1) blocks neuronal apoptosis induced by LK in cultured rat cerebellar granule neurons (D'Mello et al., 1993). This finding is particularly interesting since IGF-1 may be expressed in cerebellar Purkinje cells and may serve as a retrograde growth factor controlling granule neuron survival during cerebellar development. Conceivably, the release of IGF-1 from Purkinje cell dendrites may prevent the elimination of granule neurons via apoptosis and thus, account for the precise ratio of Purkinje cells: granule neurons observed in the adult cerebellum (Ito, 1984a).

7. G Proteins Bidirectionally Affect Apoptosis of Cerebellar Granule Neurons

Despite the impressive number of genes that have now been shown to either induce or block apoptosis, little is known about the signal transduction mechanisms which invariably precede the transcriptional events underlying apoptosis. Since we have found that both slow and fast neurotransmitters display antiapoptotic effects on cultured cerebellar granule neurons and since metabotropic glutamate and muscarinic-cholinergic receptors are coupled to G proteins, we further examined whether G proteins directly regulate apoptosis of cultured cerebellar granule neurons. Activation of specific G proteins robustly and bidirectionally affects apoptosis of cultured cerebellar granule neurons (Yan et al., 1995c). Stimulation of Gs with cholera toxin (CTX) (Gilman, 1987), for example, completely blocks apoptosis induced by nondepolarizing concentrations (5 mM) of K^+ (Fig. 6). However, pretreatment with pertussis toxin (PTX) is without effect on cerebellar granule neuron viability under any condition studied, (suggesting that a PTX-insensitive G protein(s) is involved). By contrast, stimulation of Go/Gi with the wasp venom peptide mastoparan induces apoptosis of cerebellar granule neurons even in high (depolarizing) concentrations of K^+ (Fig. 6). Moreover, pretreatment of cerebellar granule neurons with cholera toxin attenuates neuronal death induced by mastoparan (Yan et al., 1995c). However, in our hands, pertussis toxin, cell permeable analogs of cAMP, and activators of protein kinase A do not affect apoptosis of cultured cerebellar granule neurons. These data suggest that G-proteins may function as key switches for controlling the programmed death of mammalian neurons, especially in the developing central nervous system (Yan et al., 1995c).

8. Cultured Cerebellar Granule Neurons as a Model for Studying Exogenous or Endogenous Neurotoxins and Neurodegeneration

There is increasing evidence that apoptosis not only mediates the selective loss of various cell types during development, but may also mediate the pathological death of neurons induced by various toxic insults (Meyaard et al., 1992; Murakami et al., 1993; Gougeon and Montagnier, 1993).

Diphenylhydantoin (DPH), one of the most commonly prescribed anticonvulsants for the treatment of various seizure disorders (Rall and Schleifer, 1990), can also produce CNS toxicity including frank neurodegeneration at high or toxic doses (Adams et al., 1990). The age-dependent systemic and CNS side-effects and toxicity of DPH have been well characterized (Rall and Schleifer, 1990). Using cultured cerebellar granule neurons, we have observed and characterized a delayed-type of neurotoxicity induced by DPH. DPH toxicity of cerebellar granule neurons is time- and concentration-dependent (Yan et al., 1995a). Morphological studies using Nomarski optics and staining with the fluorescent dye Hoechst 33258, demonstrate that DPH-induced neurotoxicity of cerebellar granule neurons is associated with cytoplasmic blebbing, heterochromatic clumping, and condensation of chromatin, which precede cell death. Unlike glutamate toxicity (excitotoxicity), DPH-induced neurotoxicity of cerebellar granule neurons is attenuated by actinomycin D and cycloheximide, and is associated with nucleosomal-sized DNA fragmentation. Since we have previously found that depolarization of cultured cerebellar granule neurons with high concentrations of K^+ promotes the survival of these neurons by blocking apoptosis (Yan et al., 1994), we examined the effects of DPH on the K^+-evoked increase in intracellular $[Ca^{2+}]_i$. Using fura-2 microfluorimetry to measure $[Ca^{2+}]_i$ we found that neurotoxic concentrations of DPH markedly reduce the increase in $[Ca^{2+}]_i$ associated with elevated $[K^+]_e$. Taken together, these data demonstrate that exposure of cultured cerebellar granule neurons to pharmacologically-relevant concentrations of DPH results in a delayed type of neurotoxicity characterized by the biochemical and morphological features of apoptosis (Yan et al., 1995a).

Bilirubin, a degradation product of protoporphyrins derived from hemoglobin, is also a well known neurotoxin. However, the cellular and molecular mechanisms underlying bilirubin neurotoxicity are poorly described. Recently, we have found that low micromolar concentrations of bilirubin are toxic to cultured rat cerebellar granule neurons (Yan et al., 1995b). By contrast, only higher concentrations of bilirubin are toxic to cultured fetal rat cortical or hippocampal neurons. Moreover, bilirubin-induced neurotoxicity of cerebellar neurons is associated with the biochemical and morphological features of apoptosis. Further, bilirubin-induced apoptosis of cerebellar granule neurons and Purkinje cells is blocked by RNA and protein synthesis inhibitors, suggesting a gene-directed mechanism. Using gel shift (EMSA) analysis we have recently found that bilirubin activates the transcription factor NF-κB in a concentration- and time-dependent manner in cultured cerebellar granule neurons (Yan et al., 1995b). Moreover, TPCK and TLCK, proteinase inhibitors of NF-κB activation, block both bilirubin-induced apoptosis of cerebellar granule neurons and bilirubin-induced NF-κB activation. Activation of NF-κB may be an early intracellular event mediating bilirubin-induced apoptosis of cerebellar granule neurons (Yan et al., 1995b).

Summary

Cultured cerebellar granule neurons can be readily maintained in vitro in relatively homogenous primary culture. The latter requires depolarization with either elevated $[K^+]e$ or exposure to excitatory amino acid receptor agonists. Exposure to nondepolarizing culture conditions results in a time-dependent loss of neuronal viability. The death of cultured cerebellar granule neurons exposed to nondepolarizing culture condition is apoptotic in nature as ascertained by both morphological and biochemical criteria. Cultured cerebellar granule neurons represent a fascile in vitro model of neuronal apoptosis and should prove useful in elucidating the signaling and transcriptional events underlying apoptosis of neurons which occurs during normal development and/or following pathological or toxic CNS insult.

Acknowledgments

The work represented in this review are taken substantially from our previously published work (cf. Yan et al., 1994, 1995a–d).

References

Adams J., Vorheers C. V., and Middaugh L. D. (1990) Developmental neurotoxicity of anticonvulsants: human and animal evidence on phenytoin. *Neurotoxicol. Teratol.* **12,** 203–214.

Aloso R., Didier M., and Soubrie P. (1990) [³H] N-methylscopolamine binding studies reveal M2 and M3 muscarinic receptor subtypes on cerebellar granule cells in primary culture. *J. Neurochem.* **55,** 334–337.

Altman J (1972) Postnatal development of the cerebellar cortex in the rat. 3. maturation of the components of the granule layer. *J. Comp. Neurol.* **145,** 465–513.

Balázs R., Jorgensen O. S., and Hack N. (1988) N-methyl-D-aspartate promotes the survival of cerebellar granule cells in culture. *Neuroscience* **27,** 437–451.

Barinaga M. (1993) Death gives birth to the nervous system but how? *Science* **259,** 762,763.

Burgoyne R. D. and Cambray-Deakin M. A. (1988) The cellular neurobiology of neuronal development: the cerebellar granule cell. *Brain Res.* **472,** 77–101.

Cohen J. J. and Duke R. C. (1984) Glucocorticoid activation of a calcium-dependent endonuclease in thymocyte nuclei leads to cell death. *J. Immunol.* **32,** 38–42.

Copani A., Bruno M. G., Barresi V., Battaglia G., Condorelli D. F., and Nicoletti F. (1995) Activation of metabotropic glutamate receptors prevents neuronal apoptosis in culture. *J. Neurochem.* **64,** 101–108.

Courtney M. J., Lambert J. J., and Nicholls D. G. (1990) The interactions between plasma membrane depolarization and glutamate receptor activation in the regulation of cytoplasmic free calcium in cultured cerebellar granule cells. *J. Neurosci.* **10,** 3873–3879.

D'Mello S. R., Gall C., Ciotti T., and Calissano P. (1993) Induction of apoptosis in cerebellar granule neurons by low potassium: inhibition of death by insulin-like growth factor I and cAMP. *Proc. Natl. Acad. Sci. USA.* **90,** 10,989–10,993.

Fukamauchi F., Saunders P. L., Hough C., and Chuang D.-M. (1993) Agonist-induced down-regulation and antagonist-induced up-regulation of m2- and m3-muscarinic acetylcholine receptor mRNA and protein in cultured cerebellar granule cells. *Mol. Pharmacol.* **44,** 940–949.

Gallo V., Kingsbury A., Balázs R., and Jorgensen O. S. (1987) The role of depolarization in the survival and differentiation of cerebellar granule cells in culture. *J. Neurosci.* **7,** 2203–2213.

Garthwaite J., Garthwaite G., and Hajos F. (1986) Amino acid neurotoxicity: relationship to neuronal depolarization in rat cerebellar slices. *Neuroscience* **18,** 449–460.

Gilman A. G. (1987) G proteins, transducers of receptor-generated signals. *Annu. Rev. Biochem.* **56,** 615–649.

Gougeon M. L. and Montagnier L. (1993) Apoptosis in AIDS. *Science* **260,** 1269,1270.

Ito M. (1984a) Granule cells, in *The Cerebellum and Neural Control* (Ito M., ed.), Raven, New York, pp. 74–85.

Ito M. (1984b) Mossy fiber system, reticular and pontine nuclei, in *The Cerebellum and Neural Control* (Ito M., ed.), Raven, New York, pp. 235–255.

Koike T., Martin D. P., and Johnson E. M. Jr. (1989) Role of Ca^{2+} channels in the ability of membrane depolarization to prevent neuronal death induced by trophic-factor deprivation: evidence that levels of internal Ca^{2+} determine nerve growth factor dependence of sympathetic ganglion cells. *Proc. Natl. Acad. Sci. USA* **86**, 6421–6425.

Lindenboim L., Pinkas-Kramarski R., Sokolovsky M., and Stein R. (1995) Activation of muscarinic receptors inhibits apoptosis in PC12M1 cells. *J. Neurochem.* **64**, 2491–2499.

Meyaard L., Otto S. A., Jonker R. R., Mijnster M. J., Keet R. P., and Miedema F. (1992) Programmed death of T cells in HIV-1 infection. *Science* **257**, 217–219.

Murakami M., Tsubata T., Okamoto M., Shimizu A., Kumagai S., Imura H., and Honjo T. (1993) Antigen-induced apoptotic death of Ly-1 B cells responsible for autoimmune disease in transgenic mice. *Nature* **355**, 77–80.

Pabreza L. A., Dhawan S., and Kellar K. J. (1991) [^{3}H] Cytisine binding to nicotinic cholinergic receptors in brain. *Mol. Pharmacol.* **39**, 9–12.

Raff M. C., Barres B. A., Burne J. F., Coles H. S., Ishizaki Y., and Jacobson M. D. (1993) Programmed cell death and the control of cell survival: lessons from the nervous system. *Science* **262**, 695–700.

Rall T. W. and Schleifer L. S. (1990) Drugs effective in the therapy of the epilepsies, in *The Pharmacological Basis of Therapeutics, 8th ed.* (Goodman L. S., Gilman A. G., Rall T. W., Nies A. S., and Taylor P., eds.), Pergamon, New York, pp. 436–462.

Schramm M., Eimerl S., and Costa E. (1990) Serum and depolarizing agents cause acute neurotoxicity in cultured cerebellar granule cells: role of the glutamate receptor responsive to N-methyl-d-aspartate. *Proc. Natl. Acad. Sci. USA* **87**, 1193–1197.

Wyllie A. H. (1980) Glucocorticoid-induced thymocyte apoptosis is associated with endogenous endonuclease activation. *Nature* **284**, 555,556.

Wyllie A. H. (1988) *ISI Atlas of Science: Immunology,* pp. 192–196.

Wyllie A. H., Beattie G. J., and Hargreaves A. D. (1981) Chromatin changes in apoptosis. *Histochem. J.* **3**, 681–692.

Yan G.-M., Irwin R. P., Lin S.-Z., Weller M., Wood K. A., and Paul S. M. (1995a) Diphenylhydantoin induces apoptotic cell death of cultured rat cerebellar granule neurons. *J. Pharmacol. Exp. Ther.* **274**, 983–990.

Yan G.-M., Lin S.-Z., Gu J., Irwin R. P., and Paul S. M. (1995b). Biliubin induces apoptosis of cerebellar neurons via activation of NF-κB. *Abstr. Soc. Neurosci.* **21**, 1892.

Yan G.-M., Lin S.-Z., Irwin R. P., and Paul S. M. (1995c) Activation of G proteins bidirectionally affects apoptosis of cultured cerebellar granule neurons. *J. Neurochem.* **65,** 2425–2431.

Yan G.-M., Lin S.-Z., Irwin R. P., and Paul S. M. (1995) Activation of muscarinic cholinergic receptors blocks apoptosis of cultured cerebellar granule neurons. *Mol. Pharmacol.* **47,** 248–257.

Yan G.-M., Ni B., Weller M., Wood K. A., and Paul S. M. (1994) Depolarization or glutamate receptor activation blocks apoptotic cell death of cultured cerebellar granule neurons. *Brain Res.* **656,** 43–51.

Yoshitatsu S., Dag K. J. E., Von Lubitz A. S., Basile M. M., Borner Lin R. C.-S., Skolnick P., and Fossom L. H. (1994) Internucleosomal DNA fragmentation in the gerbil hippocampus following forebrain ischemia. *Neurosci. Lett.* **171,** 179–182.

Optimization and Validation of RT-PCR as a Tool to Analyze Gene Expression During Apoptosis

Steven Estus

1. Gene Expression, Apoptosis, and Programmed Cell Death

Apoptosis is a mode of cell death that has been defined largely on the basis of morphology (Wyllie et al., 1980; Clarke, 1990). The primary criteria used to delineate cell death as "apoptotic" are the condensation of nuclear chromatin and the fragmentation of nuclear DNA into oligonucleosomal-sized fragments (multiples of about 180 bp). After the stimulus that initiates cell death, cells undergoing apoptosis typically show few early morphological alterations. The polyribosomes then disintegrate and may form semicrystalline arrays concurrent with decreased global protein synthesis. The cell atrophies, but mitochondria and other organelles remain physically intact. Cells transiently show blebbing of the plasma membrane. Subsequent to the nuclear changes described above, cytoplasmic organelles start to degenerate and both nucleus and cytoplasm become compartmentalized into membrane-bound apoptotic bodies that are engulfed by phagocytic cells in intact tissues. A common, but not universal, characteristic of apoptosis is its dependence on continued RNA and protein synthesis.

The death of neurons by apoptosis contributes to physiologically appropriate neuronal loss during development and

From: *Neuromethods, Vol. 29: Apoptosis Techniques and Protocols*
Ed: J. Poirier Humana Press Inc.

to physiologically inappropriate neuronal loss in pathologic conditions. Regarding the former, maturation of the nervous system involves a sculpting process wherein approximately half of all neurons born during neurogenesis die, in a process frequently termed "programmed cell death" (PCD). Neurons "compete" for sufficient amounts of trophic factor support during their initial functional contact with target tissues; those neurons that are less successful receive inadequate quantities and die (Oppenheim, 1991). The PCD process culminates in apoptosis. That neuronal apoptosis also contributes to inappropriate neuronal loss is suggested by several lines of evidence. For example, several reports examining the incidence of neurons manifesting fragmented chromatin suggest that apoptosis contributes to cellular loss in Alzheimer's disease (Su et al., 1994; Lassmann et al., 1995) and Huntington disease (Portera-Calliau et al., 1995). Although controversial (Migheli et al., 1994), these data suggest that apoptosis likely contributes to human neurodegenerative disease. Apoptosis is also implicated as contributing to neuronal death after stroke because, in both focal and global models of ischemia, neuronal loss is accompanied by DNA fragmentation and reduced by protein synthesis inhibitors (Goto et al., 1990; Shigeno, 1990; Linnik et al., 1993; MacManus et al., 1993; MacManus et al., 1994). Apoptosis has also been associated with epilepsy in that DNA fragmentation accompanies neuronal death found in kainic acid-induced epileptic seizure models (Pollard et al., 1994).

That a genetic program underlies mammalian apoptosis, especially within the context of PCD, is supported by four sets of studies. First, RNA and protein synthesis inhibitors delay or block neuronal PCD in vitro (Martin et al., 1988) and in vivo (Oppenheim et al., 1990), as well as in certain other models of PCD (reviewed in Freeman et al., 1993), suggesting that PCD is dependent on macromolecular synthesis. This interpretation of these data is confounded by the findings that apoptosis *per se* can also be induced in neurons by the kinase inhibitor staurosporine, even in the presence of protein synthesis inhibitors (Jacobson et al., 1994), and that these macromolecular synthesis inhibitors may also have indirect effects (Ratan et al., 1994). The clearest interpretation of currently available data is that apoptosis represents the final stage of PCD; PCD, but not apoptosis, is dependent on macromolecular synthesis. The second line of evidence suggesting that cell death results from a genetic program is that the overexpression of certain genes causes apoptosis, e.g., *c-myc* in quiescent fibroblasts (Evan et al., 1992), whereas, the overexpression of other genes block apoptosis, e.g., bcl-2 blocks the death of superior cervical ganglion (SCG) neurons after NGF deprivation (Garcia et al., 1992). By indicating that pharmacologic manipulation of gene expression leads to instances wherein gene induction alters apoptosis, these data suggest the possibility of parallel endogenous programs. Third, recent work in *Drosophila* has identified a gene referred to as *reaper* that is induced in cells prior to apoptosis and is both necessary and sufficient for apoptosis (White et al., 1994); this suggests by analogy the existence of a similar, although likely more complex, genetic control of mammalian cell death. Last, we and others have identified several genes as induced in sympathetic neurons undergoing PCD caused by nerve growth factor (NGF) deprivation (Estus et al., 1994; Freeman et al., 1994; Ham et al., 1995). Moreover, the protein product of one of these induced genes, c-Jun, appears necessary for death (Estus et al., 1994; Ham et al., 1995) and, at least under certain circumstances, sufficient for death (Ham et al., 1995). Taken together, these data support the hypothesis that PCD results from the activation of a genetic program that culminates in the activation of proximate "killer" proteins or "thanatins" and, thereby, apoptosis (Johnson et al., 1989).

Previously, we wished to screen for known genes that may be induced in rat sympathetic neurons undergoing NGF deprivation-induced apoptosis. This required a quantitative and extremely sensitive technique because of the limited amounts of tissues, and, thereby RNA available. We and others have previously analyzed mRNA levels by using a technique based on PCR amplification of reverse-transcribed RNA (RT-PCR). Here, we report the optimization and validation of this method to quantify gene expression during apoptosis.

2. Materials and Methods

2.1. Materials

Mouse NGF was prepared by the method of Bocchini and Angeletti (1969). Radiochemicals were purchased from Amersham (Arlington Heights, IL). Unless otherwise stated, remaining chemicals were obtained from Sigma (St. Louis, MO).

2.2. Cell Culture

Primary cultures of sympathetic neurons were prepared from SCG of embryonic d 21 rats, as described previously (Martin et al., 1988), except that the nonneuronal cells were minimized by incubating the dissociated ganglia for 3 h on plastic tissue culture dishes prior to plating onto collagen-coated 35-mm dishes (approx 5000 cells/dish). From the point of dissociation, the neurons were maintained in culture medium consisting of 90% MEM (Life Technologies, Bethesda, MD), 10% FCS (Hyclone, Logan, UT), 50 ng/mL NGF, 20 μM uridine, and 20 μM fluorodeoxyuridine; after 5–7 d in culture, the proportion of nonneuronal cells, i.e., fibroblasts and Schwann cells, was approx 2%. Neurons were deprived of NGF by replacing the NGF containing medium with the same medium except that a polyclonal goat anti-NGF antiserum was substituted for NGF.

2.3. cDNA Preparation

Primary cultures were maintained in the presence of NGF for 6 d and then deprived of NGF for the indicated intervals. Total RNA was isolated by the method of Chomczynski and Sacchi (1987) or by using a resin-based RNA purification kit (RNAeasy, Quiagen, Chatsworth, CA). Alternatively, polyA+-enriched RNA was isolated by using an oligo-dT-cellulose mRNA purification kit (QuickPrep Micro kit, Pharmacia, Uppsala, Sweden) and concentrated by coprecipitation with glycogen, all as directed by the manufacturer. In most of our work, we have used total RNA and polyA+ RNA interchangeably, although after we recognized that RNA degradation was a component of neuronal apoptosis, we have tended to use solely polyA+ RNA based on the notion that polyA+ RNA corresponds to intact, presumably functional, RNA. In our optimized protocol, half of the RNA was converted to cDNA by reverse transcription (RT) with Moloney murine leukemia virus reverse transcriptase (Superscript, Life Technologies) with random hexamers (16 µM) as primers. The 30-µL reaction contained 50 mM Tris, pH 8.3, 40 mM KCl, 6 mM MgCl$_2$, 1 mM dithiothreitol, 500 µM each dATP, dTTP, dCTP, dGTP, and 20 U RNasin (Promega, Madison, WI). After 10 min at 20°C, the samples were incubated for 50 min at 42°C and the reaction was then terminated by adding 70 µL water and heating to 94°C for 5 min. Equivalent results were obtained when the other half of the mRNA was reverse transcribed with avian myeloblastosis virus reverse transcriptase (Promega). In optimization experiments, we compared random hexamers (16 µM) vs oligo-dT$_{12-18}$ (100 µM) as primers and also the effect of various RT temperatures; after the RT, the samples were subjected to PCR analysis. We also examined whether varying amounts of input mRNA or random hexamers altered the length or quantity of first-strand cDNA products; these products, which were radiolabeled by including 5 µCi of α-[^{32}P]-dCTP (3000 Ci/mmol) in each RT reaction, were separated by denaturing electrophoresis on 1% agarose gels. The gels were dried and the cDNA visualized by autoradiography.

2.4. PCR Analysis

For PCR amplification of specific cDNAs, stock reactions (50 µL) were prepared on ice and contained 50 µM dCTP, 100 µM dGTP, 100 µM dATP, and 100 µM dTTP, 10 µCi α-[^{32}P]-dCTP (3000 Ci/mmol), 1.5 mM MgCl$_2$ 50 mM KCl, 10 mM Tris, pH 9.0, 0.1% Triton X-100, 1 µM each primer, 1 U of Taq polymerase, and 3% of the cDNA synthesized in the RT reaction. Primer sequences for cyclophilin, neurofilament M (NF-M), tyrosine hydroxylase (TOH), and S100β have been

Table 1
PCR Primer Sequences

Gene	Primer	Sequence	Reference
Transglutaminase	5'	ACAGGAGAAGAGCGAAGGGA	Gentile
	3'	TTGACCTCGGCAAACACGAA	et al., 1991
TGFβ1	5'	ACCGGCCTCCCGCAAAGACTT	Tsuji et al., 1990
	3'	GGAAGCTATTGCCAGCAGGT	
Calmodulin	5'	GCAGAGCTGCAGGACATGAT	Nojima
	3'	TCCTTATCAAACACACCGGAA	et al., 1987
C-FOS	5'	AATAAGATGGCTGCAGCCAA	Curran
	3'	TTGGCAATCTCGGTCTGCAA	et al., 1987
HSC73	5'	GGCCAAGCGCACCCTCTCCT	Sorger and
	3'	ATTCAGCTCTTTTCCATTGA	Pelham, 1987
HSP70	5'	GCCCAAGGTGCAGGTGAAC	Longo
	3'	CGTGATCACCGCGTTGGTCA	et al., 1993

published previously (Freeman et al., 1994). Further oligo sequences are presented in Table 1. The stock solutions were separated into three equal aliquots, covered with a drop of mineral oil, and subjected to various numbers of PCR cycles to determine the minimum number of cycles necessary to detect the PCR product. The typical reaction conditions were 1 min at 95°C, 1 min at 55°C, and 2 min at 72°C. We found that the number of PCR cycles required to generate detectable cDNA product does not necessarily correlate well with the abundance of the original mRNA; whereas the efficiency of RT-PCR is typically quite consistent for a given RNA and primer pair, RT efficiency can vary between RNAs because of variability in RNA secondary structure and between primers because of amplification efficiency. Therefore, the data presented should be taken to be indicative of changes in the abundance of mRNAs between samples and only a rough indication of absolute mRNA levels. After amplification, the cDNAs were separated by electrophoresis on 12% polyacrylamide gels, visualized by autoradiography of the dried gels, and quantified by excising the radioactive bands from the gel by using the autoradiogram as a template, or more recently, by using a PhosphorImager (Molecular Dynamics, Sunnyvale, CA). Prior to drying, the gels were stained with ethidium bromide to allow visualization of molecular weight markers (1 kb ladder, Life Technologies); these markers are visualized after drying by holding the gels tangential to a UV light box.

The identity of the cDNA amplified by each primer pair was confirmed by either direct sequencing (Promega, fmole sequencing kit), by subcloning the amplified cDNAs into pBluescript (Stratagene, La Jolla, CA), or, more recently and more efficiently, by subcloning with the TA cloning kit (Invitrogen, San Diego, CA), and then sequencing the inserts. Of some 50 odd PCR products that have been sequenced to date, only two have proven to be derived from incorrect genes. The linearity of the RT-PCR technique was assessed by pooling RNA from control and NGF deprived cultures, subjecting various quantities to RT, and then 3% of the resultant cDNA to PCR.

3. Results

3.1. Optimization of RT-PCR Assay

Screening scores of genes to identify patterns of gene expression in dying cells is hampered in many model systems by the limiting numbers of cells and hence quantities of RNA available. To facilitate such an analysis, we optimized a quantitative, extremely sensitive, PCR-based technique. In brief, mRNA was converted to cDNA, portions of which were then subjected to limited numbers of cycles of PCR amplification in the presence of specific oligo pairs and α-[^{32}P]-dCTP; the resulting radiolabeled cDNA products were then separated by gel electrophoresis, and visualized and quantified by subjecting the dried gel to autoradiography and PhosphorImager analysis. In optimizing this assay, we examined several reaction parameters. First, we assessed whether

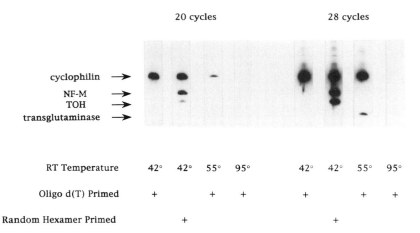

Fig. 1. Random hexamer priming of RNA produces a more complete cDNA pool than oligo-dT priming. Neuronal RNA was subjected to RT with either random hexamers or oligo-dT as primers as described in Section 2. Equivalent proportions of the reaction products were then subjected to 20 or 28 cycles of PCR to examine the levels of the indicated mRNAs. The effects of RT temperature were also examined; the quantities of PCR products resulting when the RT was performed at 20°C for 10 min and then either 42°C or 55°C for 50 min, or only 95°C for 10 min, are depicted.

random hexamers or oligo-dT priming of the RT generated a more representative first-strand cDNA pool (Fig. 1). Identical samples of neuronal RNA were reverse transcribed by using either random hexamers or oligo-dT as primers. Equivalent proportions of the reaction products were then subjected to 20 or 28 cycles of PCR. Whereas the yields of the PCR-amplified cDNA corresponding to *cyclophilin* were equivalent with random hexamer or oligo-dT primed cDNA, yields of cDNA corresponding to *neurofilament-M (NF-M)* or *tyrosine hydroxylase (TOH)* were much decreased in the oligo-dT-primed sample (compare yields at 20 cycles, 42°C RT temperature). The decreased efficiency of oligo-dT priming for these mRNAs was attributed to the fact that the nucleotides intervening between their polyA tail and the sequences that were PCR amplified were too numerous for highly efficient reverse transcription, i.e., these distances were approx 1580 bp for *TOH* and approx 2450 bp for *NF-M*, compared with only approx 500 bp for *cyclophilin*. Since the utility of random hexamers appears relatively independent of the distance between the amplified region and the polyA tail, we recommend their use for routine quantitative RT-PCR.

We also examined the effects of varying the RT temperature; we noted that temperatures that decreased RNA secondary structure, e.g., 55°C, dramatically decreased overall cDNA yields (Fig. 1, compare cyclophilin yields after 20 cycles). However, these higher temperatures were required for the detection of RNAs with apparent high levels of secondary structure, e.g., transglutaminase (Fig. 1, compare transglutaminase band at 55°C vs no band present at 42°C RT). This observation emphasizes the necessity of positive controls to ensure that the absence of PCR product is reflective of the absence of gene expression. To confirm that the cDNA products were derived from RNA and not contaminating genomic DNA or PCR products, we also examined 95°C as an RT temperature; as would be expected, no cDNA was detected.

In optimizing reaction conditions, we also examined the effect of various concentrations of RNA or random hexamer on cDNA yield and length. The cDNAs were radiolabeled during the RT by including α-[^{32}P]-dCTP in the reaction and were then separated by denaturing gel electrophoresis. The quantities of cDNA were proportional to the quantities of input RNA (Fig. 2). The size of the cDNA, which averaged 1 kbp, was independent of input RNA. The effect of altering random hexamer concentrations was more complex: Lower concentrations of random hexamer produced longer cDNAs but at lower yields (Fig. 2). This probably indicates that random hexamers at low concentrations bind to RNA with a greater spacing than at high concentrations, allowing the reverse transcriptase to transcribe longer lengths of RNA. Lastly, we examined the effects of glycogen on the RT reaction because we use glycogen as a "carrier" to precipitate the small amounts of polyA+ RNA obtained from the SCG neurons. Total RNA from PC12 cells (1 µg) was reverse transcribed in the presence or absence of 100 µg of glycogen.

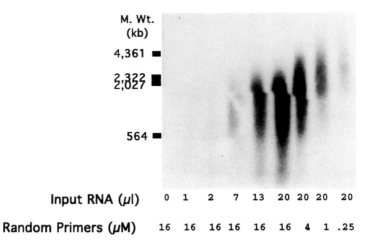

Fig. 2. Relationship between first strand cDNA synthesis and various concentrations of RNA and random hexamers is shown. RNA was reverse transcribed in the presence of α-[^{32}P]-d-CTP and the resultant cDNA separated by denaturing gel electrophoresis. Varying the quantities of input RNA resulted in proportional changes in first-strand cDNA yield, but had no effect on the lengths of the first-strand cDNAs. Decreasing random hexamer concentrations increased the lengths of first-strand cDNA, but decreased overall cDNA yields.

Glycogen appeared to have no inhibitory effect on RT efficiency (data not shown).

In summary, the average cDNA length produced by the RT reaction was approx 1 kbp. To ensure that the length of the cDNA fragments amplified by PCR is much less than the length of the first strand cDNA, we typically amplify cDNA fragments in the range of 60–200 bp. By using the technique described here, the yields of cDNA generated from the RNA of approx 5000 neurons were sufficient for 60 PCR reactions.

3.2. Validation of RT-PCR Assay

To assess the quantitative reliability of this optimized RT-PCR assay, we have performed two validation tests. First, we examined whether the output of PCR products was linearly proportional to the input RNA. PCR amplification can be modeled by the relationship

$$cDNA_n = cDNA_0(1+E)n$$

in which $cDNA_n$ is the quantity of cDNA product after n cycles; $cDNA_0$ is the initial quantity of cDNA; and E is the amplification efficiency ($0 < E < 1$). Hence, if the amplification efficiency is unaltered during the amplification, the quantity of PCR product is linearly proportional to the quantity of initial cDNA. Moreover, if the RNA is the limiting reagent in the RT, the initial cDNA quantities are proportional to the input RNA. By using the minimal numbers of PCR cycles necessary to detect the cDNAs, we found that the yields of PCR products were linearly proportional to input RNA (Fig. 3). Hence, this assay could be useful in providing an indication of changes in the relative quantities of a given mRNA.

The second critical aspect we examined was whether RT-PCR could be used to detect the induction of a specific gene and, for these experiments, we used a well-established paradigm, i.e., the induction of the 70-kDa heat-shock protein, HSP70. Sympathetic primary neurons were maintained in vitro for 6 d, and then subjected to a 44°C heat shock for 30 min. RNA was isolated 3- and 24-h later, and the levels of specific mRNAs were compared with those in a parallel control sample. A robust induction of *HSP70* was observed in neuronal RNA 3 h, but not 24 h, after the heat shock (Fig. 4). No significant changes were seen in mRNAs encoding the constitutively expressed genes *cyclophilin* and *HSC73* (another member of the HSP family), or *TGFβ1* (Fig. 4). Hence, RT-PCR can be used successfully to detect changes in the expression of a specific gene.

3.3. Application of RT-PCR Assay

In initial work examining gene expression during apoptosis by using RT-PCR, we isolated total RNA from neurons deprived of NGF for various intervals, quantified the RNA yields, and then used constant amounts of RNA in RT-PCR reactions. When we compared the expression patterns of a neuronal marker, TOH, and a nonneuronal marker, S100b, we found that NGF deprivation was associated with

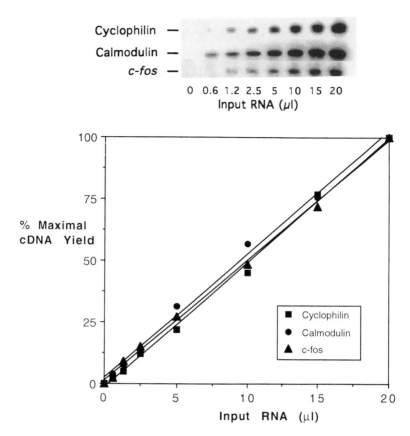

Fig. 3. Linearity of RT-PCR assay with input mRNA: Varying quantities of a stock of neuronal polyA+ RNA were reverse transcribed and subjected to PCR amplification in the presence of specific primer pairs as described in Section 2. The resultant cDNAs were separated by PAGE and incorporated radioactivity was determined by PhosphorImager analysis.

decreasing levels of TOH mRNA and increasing levels of S100 mRNA (Fig. 5). Hence, the nonneuronal marker appeared to be induced during neuronal apoptosis. On reflection, we recognized that as apoptosis proceeded, the contribution of neuronal RNA to the isolated RNA decreased, with nonneuronal RNA making up the difference. Hence, in our subsequent work, we normalized our RT-PCR analyses to the numbers of cells originally plated, i.e., we used a constant proportion

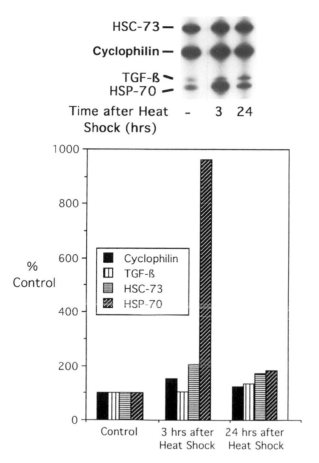

Fig. 4. Detection of altered gene expression with RT-PCR is shown. Primary neuronal cultures were maintained in the presence of NGF for 6 d, placed at 44°C for 30 min, and allowed to recover for 3 or 24 h. RNA was then isolated and subjected to RT-PCR. The upper panel depicts a typical RT-PCR result, whereas the graphical data represent the averages of two separate determinations.

of isolated RNA for RT-PCR analyses. When we applied this approach, the amounts of nonneuronal RNA remained constant during neuronal apoptosis, allowing us to more easily identify genes that were actually induced (Estus et al., 1994; Freeman et al., 1994). These results also suggest the practicality of using *in situ* hybridization or immunohistochemis-

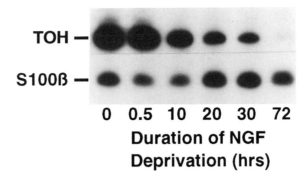

Fig. 5. Normalization of RT-PCR to input RNA may lead to ambiguous results. Primary neuronal cultures were maintained in the presence of NGF for 6 d. The cultures were then deprived of NGF and, after the indicated intervals, total RNA isolated (Chomczynski and Sacchi, 1987). After the RNA was quantified by UV absorption, 1-µg aliquots were reverse transcribed and 3% portions of the resulting cDNA subjected to PCR analysis.

try to directly demonstrate that gene expression originates from the expected cell type in studies involving heterogeneous cell populations.

4. Discussion

4.1. Overview

In this report, we have described experiments that were directed towards the optimization and validation of quantitative RT-PCR. Moreover, the TOH/S100β comparison serves as a demonstration of a possible source of interpretative error. Based on our experience, we have concluded that in situations involving the need to analyze multiple genes and in which only very small quantities of RNA are available, RT-PCR appears the technique of choice because of its sensitivity and reliability. We also want to emphasize that these results were obtained by using the minimal number of PCR cycles that were necessary to detect the radioactive product. In general, the quantities of these PCR products that were quantified by radioactivity were not sufficient to discern by ethidium bromide staining.

4.2. RT-PCR Quantitation of Gene Expression

A variety of RT-PCR-based approaches have been proposed for the analysis of gene expression (reviewed in Foley et al., 1993). The major difference among these approaches is whether RNA is measured in an absolute or relative sense. To measure absolute quantities of RNA optimally requires the use of an internal RNA standard that is specific for the gene of interest because the efficiency of RT-PCR varies in a gene-and primer-specific fashion. Alternatively, RT-PCR as described here appears well suited to compare relative levels of specific mRNAs among multiple samples that are otherwise quite similar. For example, in the heat shock study described here, we compared relative levels of mRNA between treated and nontreated cultures. The demonstration that HSP70 mRNA was increased was facilitated by identifying reference genes that were not induced. The primary requirement for validating this approach was that the PCR product yields were linear with respect to input RNA, a requirement that was satisfied in initial validation studies. Moreover, in work published elsewhere (Estus et al., 1994; Freeman et al., 1994), we have confirmed that genes identified as induced by RT-PCR are actually induced, as detected by using *in situ* hybridization analyses. Hence, the RT-PCR-based assay described here has facilitated a reliable and quantitative analysis of gene expression.

The reliance of this research on RT-PCR is made even more significant by recognizing that such analyses would not have been feasible by using more standard techniques. For example, starting with approx 5000 SCG neurons, we isolated RNA equivalent to 0.1 μg of total RNA, and generated cDNA sufficient for 60 PCR analyses. In contrast to this level of sensitivity, typical ribonuclease protection or Northern blot assays require on the order of 10 times this quantity of RNA to examine the expression of far fewer genes. Hence, since only approx 10,000 SCG neurons are obtained from each rat fetus, the examination of multiple genes by other techniques would have required a prohibitive numbers of animals.

In summary, this application of RT-PCR has two primary properties. First, the exquisite sensitivity of the technique allows the examination of many different mRNAs in small quantities of RNA. Second, whereas the results obtained with the technique provide limited information about absolute mRNA levels, changes in the relative expression of specific genes are easily identifiable.

Acknowledgments

We thank members of the Eugene Johnson laboratory at Washington University (namely Robert Freeman and Eugene Johnson) as well as the Steven Younkin laboratory at Case Western Reserve University (namely Todd Golde, Linda Younkin, and Steven Younkin) for their critical insights into the development of this RT-PCR technique. The experiments described here were performed by S. E. during postdoctoral work in the Johnson laboratory. We also thank P. A. Lampe, J. L. Colombo, and P. A. K. Osborne for their expert technical assistance, and P. A. K. Osborne, Michael Tucker, and Eugene Johnson for critically reviewing this manuscript. This work was supported by a French Foundation for Alzheimer's Research fellowship (S. E.), NIH training grants HL07275 (S. E.), and grants from the Washington University School of Medicine Alzheimer's Disease Research Center (P50–AG05681), and the American Paralysis Association.

References

Chomczynski P. and Sacchi N. (1987) Single-step method of RNA isolation by acid guanidinium thiocyanate-phenol-chloroform extraction. *Anal. Biochem.* **162,** 156–159.

Clarke P. G. (1990) Developmental cell death: morphological diversity and multiple mechanisms. *Anat. Embryol. (Berl).* **181(3),** 195–213.

Curran T., Gordon M. B., Rubino K. L., and Sambucetti L. C. (1987) Isolation and characterization of the c-fos (rat) cDNA and analysis of post translational modification in vitro. *Oncogene* **2,** 79–84.

Estus S., Zaks W., Freeman R., Gruda M., Bravo R., and Johnson E. (1994) Altered gene expression in neurons during programmed cell death; identification of c-jun as necessary for neuronal apoptosis. *J. Cell Biol.* **127,** 1717–1727.

Evan G. I., Wyllie A. H., Gilbert C. S., Littlewood T. D., Land H., Brooks M., Waters C. M., Penn L. Z., and Hancock D. C. (1992) Induction of apoptosis in fibroblasts by *c-myc* protein. *Cell* **69(1)**, 119–128.

Foley K. P., Leonard M. W., and Engel J. E. (1993) Quantitation of RNA using the polymerase chain reaction. *Trends Genet.* **9**, 381–384.

Freeman R. S., Estus S., Horigome K., and Johnson E. M., Jr. (1993) Cell death genes in invertebrates and (maybe) vertebrates. *Curr. Opin. Neurobiol.* **3(1)**, 25–31.

Freeman R. S., Estus S., and Johnson E. M., Jr. (1994) Analysis of cell cycle-related gene expression in postmitotic neurons: selective induction of cyclin D1 during programmed cell death. *Neuron* **12**, 343–355.

Garcia I., Martinou I., Tsujimoto Y., and Martinou J.-C. (1992) Prevention of programmed cell death of sympathetic neurons by the bcl-2 proto-oncogene. *Science* **258**, 302–304.

Gentile V., Saydak M., Chiocca E. A., Akande O., Birckbichler P. J., Lee K. N., Stein J. P., and Davies P. J. A. (1991) Isolation and characterization of cDNA clones to mouse macrophage and human endothelial cell tissues transglutaminases. *J. Biol. Chem.* **266**, 478–483.

Goto K., Ishige A., Sekiguchi K., Iizuka S., Sugimoto A., and Yuzurihara M. (1990) Effects of cycloheximide on delayed neuronal death in rat hippocampus. *Brain Res.* **534**, 299–302.

Ham J., Babij C., Whitfield J., Pfarr C. M., Lallemand D., Yaniv M., and Rubin L. L. (1995) A c-Jun dominant negative mutant protects sympathetic neurons against programmed cell death. *Neuron* **14**, 927–939.

Jacobson M. D., Burne J. F., and Raff M. C. (1994) Programmed cell death and Bcl-2 protection in the absence of a nucleus. *EMBO J.* **13**, 1899–1910.

Johnson E. M., Chang J. Y., Koike T., and Martin D. P. (1989) Why do neurons die when deprived of trophic factor? *Neurobiol. Aging* **10**, 549–552.

Lassmann H., Bancher C., Breitschopf H., Wegiel J., Bobinski M., Jellinger K., and Wisniewski H. M. (1995) Cell death in Alzheimer's disease evaluated by DNA fragmentation *in situ*. *Acta Neuropathol. (Berl.)* **89**, 35–41.

Linnik M. D., Zobrist R. H., and Hatfield M. D. (1993) Evidence supporting a role for programmed cell death in focal cerebral ischemia in rats. *Stroke* **24**, 2002–2009.

Longo F. M., Wang S., Narasimhan P., Zhang J. S., Chen J., Massa S. M., and Sharp F. R. (1993) cDNA cloning and expression of stress-inducible rat hsp70 in normal and injured rat brain. *J. Neurosci. Res.* **36**, 325–335.

MacManus J. P., Buchan A. M., Hill I. E., Rasquinha I., and Preston E. (1993) Global ischemia can cause DNA fragmentation indicative of apoptosis in rat brain. *Neurosci. Lett.* **164**, 89–92.

MacManus J. P., Hill I. E., Huang Z. G., Rasquinha I., Xue D., and Buchan A. M. (1994) DNA damage consistent with apoptosis in transient ischaemic neocortex. *NeuroReport* **5**, 493–496.

Martin D. P., Schmidt R. E., DiStefano P. S., Lowry O. H., Carter J. G., and Johnson E. M., Jr. (1988) Inhibitors of protein synthesis and RNA synthesis prevent neuronal death caused by nerve growth factor deprivation. *J. Cell Biol.* **106(3)**, 829–844.

Migheli A., Cavalla P., Marino S., and Schiffer D. (1994) A study of apoptosis in normal and pathologic nervous tissue after *in situ* end-labeling of DNA strand breaks. *J Neuropathol. Exp. Neurol.* **53**, 606–616.

Nojima H., Kishi K., and Sokabe H. (1987) Multiple calmodulin mRNA species are derived from two distinct genes. *Mol. Cell. Biol.* **7**, 1873–1880.

Oppenheim R. W., Prevette D., Tytell M., and Homma S. (1990) Naturally occurring and induced neuronal death in the chick embryo in vivo requires protein and RNA synthesis: evidence for the role of cell death genes. *Dev. Biol.* **138(1)**, 104–113.

Pollard H., Cantagrel S., Charriaut-Marlangue C., Moreau J., and Ben Ari Y. (1994) Apoptosis associated DNA fragmentation in epileptic brain damage. *NeuroReport* **5**, 1053-1055.

Portera-Calliau C., Hedreen J. C., Price D. L., and Koliatsos V. E. (1995) Evidence for apoptotic cell death in Huntington disease and excitotoxic animal models. *J. Neurosci.* **15**, 3775–3787.

Ratan R. R., Murphy T. H., and Baraban J. M. (1994) Macromolecular synthesis inhibitors prevent oxidative stress-induced apoptosis in embryonic neurons by shunting cysteine from protein synthesis to glutathione. *J. Neurosci.* **14**, 4385–4392.

Shigeno T. (1990) Reduction of delayed neuronal death by inhibition of protein synthesis. *Neurosci. Lett.* **120**, 117–119.

Sorger P. K. and Pelham H. R. (1987) Cloning and expression of a gene encoding hsc73, the major hsp70–like protein in unstressed rat cells. *EMBO J.* **6**, 993–998.

Su J. H., Anderson A. J., Cummings B. J., and Cotman C. W. (1994) Immunohistochemical evidence for apoptosis in Alzheimer's disease. *Neuroreport* **5**, 2529–2533.

Tsuji T., Okada F., Yamaguchi K., and Nakamura T. (1990) Molecular cloning of the large subunit of transforming growth factor type beta masking protein and expression of the mRNA in various rat tissues. *Proc. Natl. Acad. Sci. USA* **87**, 8835–8839.

White K., Grether M. E., Abrams J. M., Young L., Farrell K., and Steller H. (1994) Genetic control of programmed cell death in *Drosophila*. *Science* **264**, 677–683.

Wyllie A. H., Kerr J. F. R., and Currie A. R. (1980) Cell death: the significance of apoptosis. *Int. Rev. Cytol.* **68**, 251–306.

p53 Induction Is a Marker of Neuronal Apoptosis in the Central Nervous System

Shahin Sakhi and Steven S. Schreiber

1. Apoptosis in the Central Nervous System

Apoptosis is an active process of selective cell death that occurs during development and has been implicated in the pathogenesis of a variety of human diseases (Thompson, 1995). Apoptosis can be distinguished from the other major form of cell death, necrosis, on the basis of both morphological and biochemical features; these include chromatin condensation with nuclear pyknosis, and cytoplasmic shrinkage (Thompson, 1995). One prominent hallmark of apoptosis is a characteristic pattern of DNA cleavage into oligonucleosome-sized fragments that, under most circumstances, can be visualized by agarose gel electrophoresis. However, when relatively few apoptotic cells are present, fragmented DNA can be labeled *in situ* by more sensitive techniques. Using this approach, apoptotic cell death has been documented in the rodent central nervous system (CNS) following cerebral ischemia (Heron et al., 1993; MacManus et al., 1994), status epilepticus (Filipowski et al., 1994; Pollard et al., 1994; Sakhi et al., 1994) and adrenalectomy (Schreiber et al., 1994). Similar methods have been used to demonstrate apoptotic cells in the brain of patients with Alzheimer's (Su et al., 1994; Lassamn et al., 1995) and Huntington's diseases (Portera-Cailliau et al., 1995). Whether neuronal apoptosis plays a

From: *Neuromethods, Vol. 29: Apoptosis Techniques and Protocols*
Ed: J. Poirier Humana Press Inc.

primary role in the pathogenesis of neurologic disease, however, remains to be determined. Another major feature of apoptotic cell death is a requirement for macromolecular synthesis, implying the activation of genes encoding "killer proteins" (Steller, 1995). Apoptosis-associated genes have recently been identified in nonneural mammalian systems and during invertebrate development (Cohen, 1993; Stellar, 1995). Nonetheless, definitive evidence for cell death genes in the CNS is lacking. Upon characterization of such genes, their encoded proteins could be the potential targets of specific pharmacotherapies, and possibly lead to effective treatment of a number of devastating neurologic diseases.

2. Tumor Suppressor p53: Cell Cycle Arrest vs Cell Death

Several lines of evidence have led to the idea that terminally differentiated neurons undergo apoptosis when prompted to re-enter an aberrant cell cycle. In this regard, both apoptosis and mitosis share certain morphological features (Stellar, 1995). In addition, genes which play a role in modulating cell proliferation, such as c-*myc,* c-*fos,* c-*jun,* cyclin D1, and p53 have been implicated in apoptosis (Colatta et al., 1992; Lane, 1992; Shi et al., 1992; Schreiber et al., 1993; Smeyne et al., 1993; Dragunow et al., 1994; Freeman et al., 1994; Ham et al., 1995). In attempting to identify apoptosis-related genes in the CNS, we focused our attention on the tumor suppressor gene, p53 (Levine et al., 1991). Enormous interest in p53 has developed in recent years because of a high percentage of human malignancies that are associated with p53 mutations (Hollstein et al., 1991). The p53 gene product is a 53 kDa phosphoprotein that has sequence-specific DNA binding properties and acts as a transcription factor (Kern et al., 1991; Farmer et al., 1992). A number of studies have shown that overexpression of wild-type p53 protein arrests the cell cycle at the G1-S interphase (Kastan et al., 1991; Kuerbitz et al., 1992). Experimental evidence suggests that p53-mediated cell cycle arrest is regulated by at least on p53-inducible gene, waf1 (wild-type p53-activated fragment), a cyclin-dependent kinase inhibitor (El-Deiry et al., 1994). In addition, various DNA-damaging agents including UV and X irradiation, and chemotherapeutic drugs are known to induce p53 activity (Kastan et al., 1991; Zhan et al., 1993). Thus, p53-mediated cell cycle arrest following genomic damage is an important mechanism of cell growth control that probably facilitates DNA repair prior to replication. Under certain conditions, however, nuclear accumulation of wild-type p53 protein results in apoptosis, which can be taken as an extreme form of cell growth control. Accordingly, transfection of p53 constructs into cells that normally lack endogenous p53 expression causes apoptosis (Yonish-Rouach et al., 1991; Ryan et al., 1993). Further, p53 induction in vivo results in tumor regression in nude mice that is morphologically consistent with apoptosis (Shaw et al., 1992). These examples indicate that increased p53 expression may not only serve as a cellular marker of apoptosis, but may play an active role in the cell death process. Currently, the factors that determine whether p53 induction will lead to cell cycle arrest or cell death are poorly understood. It is likely that the phase of the cell cycle, extent of DNA damage, and cell type are all important. We, therefore, speculated that p53 overexpression in terminally differentiated neurons in the CNS might lead to neuronal apoptosis.

3. p53 Induction Is Restricted to Apoptotic Neurons Following Excitotoxin Treatment

Systemic administration of the glutamate analog, kainic acid (KA), causes a well-described seizure disorder and neuronal loss in fields CA1 and CA3 of the hippocampus, piriform cortex, amygdala, and several thalamic nuclei, yet sparing other structures,, such as the granule cell layer of the dentate gyrus (Schwab et al., 1980; Nitecka et al., 1984). Recent data, including the results of ultrastructural studies, indicate that KA-induced neuronal death is consistent with apoptosis (Filipowski et al., 1994; Pollard et al., 1994). In addition, the extent of KA-induced death is significantly attenuated by the protein synthesis inhibitor, cycloheximide, suggesting that there is a requirement for *de novo* protein synthesis (Schreiber et al., 1993). We were interested in investigating the role of p53 in KA-induced neuronal death (Sakhi et al., 1994). Adult Sprague-Dawley rats were treated systemically with KA and sacrificed at various times following the onset of seizure activity. In summary, between 4–16 h after seizure-onset, a significant increase in p53 expression was observed in KA-vulnerable regions, and was restricted to neurons that appeared to be morphologically injured, i.e., condensed chromatin, eosinophilic cytoplasm, and overall cell shrinkage (Fig. 1B, Table 1). In addition, the increase in p53 expression following KA treatment was prevented by cycloheximide (Table 1).

These results have been replicated in vitro using organotypic hippocampal slice cultures (OHC) (Sakhi et al., 1995). In these studies, the effects of either KA or *N*-methyl-D-aspartate (NMDA) on p53 mRNA expression were evaluated in cultured hippocampal explants prepared from 7-d-old rats, and grown for an additional 16–19 d. As in the in vivo model, p53 induction occurred within several hours of exposure to either drug (Fig. 2). Emulsion autoradiography revealed that p53 mRNA was elevated only in injured neurons, and was relatively low in normal appearing cells (not shown).

Since p53 induction is triggered by damage to the genome, the presence of DNA damage was evaluated by *in situ* labeling. As expected, the regional distribution of cells with fragmented DNA closely overlapped that of cells exhibiting p53 induction in vivo and in vitro (Fig. 1C, D). Interestingly, NMDA appeared to cause more extensive neuronal injury compared to KA (Sakhi et al., 1995). DNA fragmentation following in vivo KA has previously been demonstrated (Filipowski et al., 1994; Pollard et al., 1994). However, when there are relatively few apoptotic cells present, fragmented DNA can be difficult to visualize by standard agarose gel electrophoresis. *In situ* end labeling is a more sensitive tech-

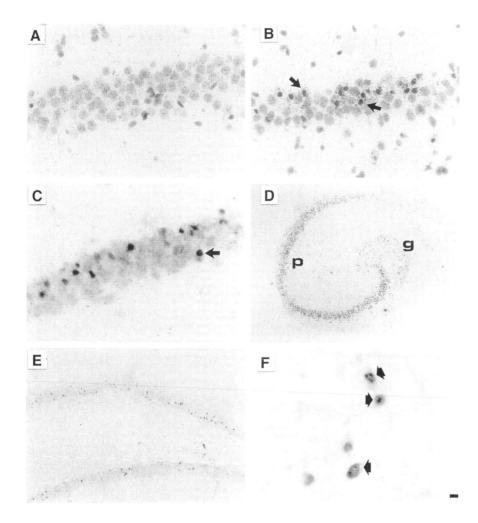

Fig. 1. p53 expression (A,B) and DNA fragmentation (C–F) in vivo and in vitro. *In situ* hybridization and emulsion autoradiography with a p53 ribo-probe was performed as described (Sakhi et al., 1994). Representative sections from the CA1 hippocampal region of a control rat **(A)** and 16 h following onset of KA-induced seizures **(B)**. Note accumulation of silver grains over cells with eosinophilic cytoplasm and condensed nucleus (arrows); hematoxylin and eosin counterstain. **(C)** *In situ* nick translation performed on an adjacent section shows the distribution of cells with fragmented DNA (e.g., arrow); hematoxylin counterstain. **(D)** DNA fragmentation in organotypic hippocampal culture treated with NMDA for 3 h, and grown for an additional 24 h. Labeled cells are present in both the pyramidal and granule cell layers. **(E)** DNA fragmentation in granule cell layer 3 d after adrenalectomy. **(F)** At high magnification, clumps of chromatin can be visualized within injured granule cells (arrowheads); acid fuchsin counterstain. Scale bar: 30 μm (A–C); 0.3 mm (D); 120 μm (E); 12 μm (F).

Table 1
Effect of Various Treatments on p53 Expression
in Hippocampal Pyramidal Cells

Treatment	Grains/500 μm^2
Control	18.0 +/− 1.3[NS]
KA	64.0 +/− 8.5[a]
CHX/KA	19.0 +/− 2.6[b]

Animals received KA (10 mg/kg, sc) with or without cycloheximide (CHX) pretreatment (2 mg/kg, sc) and were sacrificed 16 h after seizure onset. Untreated animals served as controls. *In situ* hybridization with a radiolabeled antisense p53 riboprobe and emulsion autoradiography were performed as described (Sakhi et al., 1994). Eighty cells from both the CA3 and CA1 pyramidal cell subfields were analyzed in each group (20 cells per animal, four animals per group). In the KA-treated group only those cells exhibiting cytoplasmic eosinophilia and nuclear condensation (i.e., features of cell damage) were included. Each value in the table represents the mean ± SEM Statistical analysis was performed using Student's *t*-test.
[a]$p < 0.001$ (KA vs control).
[b]$p < 0.004$ (KA vs CHX/KA).
NS: not significant (control vs CHX/KA).

nique that enables the detection of DNA damage at times earlier than would be predicted from gel electrophoresis data. Although several techniques are currently available, we prefer nick translation with DNA polymerase I, rather than end labeling with terminal transferase (i.e., TUNEL) because of a greater signal-to-noise ratio.

4. *In Situ* Nick Translation Protocol for Frozen Sections

1. Thaw sections at room temperature (RT), 4'–5'.
2. Fix sections in 4% paraformaldehyde/1X PBS, pH 7.0–7.4, RT, 10'–20'.
3. Rinse in 1X PBS, RT, 3 × 100'.
4. Rinse in H$_2$O, RT, 1'.
5. Incubate with triethanolamine (TEA), pH 8.0, RT, 1', followed by acetic anhydride/0.1M TEA, RT, 10'.

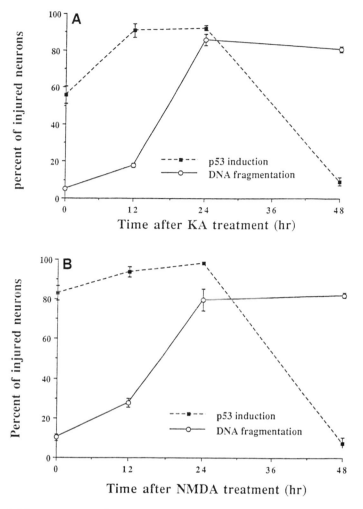

Fig. 2. Time-course of p53 induction and DNA fragmentation in excito-toxin-treated OHC. The percentage of injured neurons (i.e., total of 2500 injured neurons/group counted) exhibiting either p53 induction or DNA fragmentation was plotted as a function of time. The results are depicted as mean ± SEM for each time-point.

6. Transfer to 2X SSC, RT, 20'.
7. Dehydrate in graded ethanols and air dry.
8. Apply labeling mixture (A) to sections (generally, 50 µL/cm²) and incubate in a humid chamber, 37°C, 1 h.
9. Neutralize the reaction with 20 m*M* EDTA, pH 8.0, RT, 1'–2'.

10. Apply alkaline phosphatase-conjugated antidigoxigenin antibody (1/250 in 5% sheep serum diluted in 1X genius buffer 1, Boehringer Mannheim, Mannheim, Germany), and incubate in humid chamber with mild shaking, RT, 90'.
11. Rinse in 1X genius buffer 1, RT, 3 × 5'.
12. Rinse in 1X genius buffer 3, RT, 2 × 5'.
13. Apply chromagen mixture in the dark and check for color change every 30'.
14. Rinse in 1X genius buffer 3, RT, 2 × 5'.
15. Rinse in 1X genius buffer 4, RT, 2 × 5'.
16. Rinse in H_2O, RT, 2'.
17. Dehydrate in 70% ethanol, air dry, and coverslip using permount.
18. Labeling mixture (A):
    a. 1X nick translation buffer (10X buffer = 500 mM Tris-HCl, pH 7.2, 100 mM MgSO$_4$, 1 mM DTT).
    b. DNA labeling mixture (0.02 mM each dATP, dCTP, dGTP, 13 mM dTTP, 7 μM digoxigenin-11-dUTP, Boehringer Mannheim). Use 2 μL of DNA labeling mixture for every 100 μL of A.
    c. DNA polymerase I, endonuclease free, 10 U/100 μL (Promega, Madison, WI).
19. Chromagen mixture: To make 10 mL chromagen mixture, add the following to 1X genius buffer 3:
    a. 2.4 mg levamisol (Sigma, St. Louis, MO) to block endogenous phosphatase.
    b. 45 μL nitroblue tetrazolium (NBT, Boehringer Mannheim).
    c. 35 μL X-phosphate (Boehringer Mannheim).

5. p53 Is Induced in Apoptotic Granule Cells Following Adrenalectomy

Experimental evidence has recently shown that, following adrenalectomy (ADX), hippocampal granule cells die through an apoptotic process (Sloviter et al., 1993a,b). This provided a second model in which to investigate the relationship between p53 expression and neuronal death

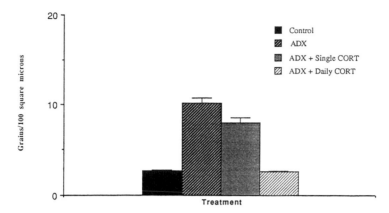

Fig. 3. Level of p53 expression in dentate gyrus granule cells. *In situ* hybridization and emulsion autoradiography with a p53 riboprobe was performed as described (Schreiber et al., 1994). Each value represents the mean ± SEM. The ADX groups are all 3 d survivals. The number of grains per unit area was significantly increased 3 d following ADX, with or without a single CORT injection, compared to unoperated controls ($p < 0.0001$). There was a significant difference in grain counts between the two ADX groups ($p < 0.02$), but no difference between adrenalectomized rats receiving daily CORT replacement and unoperated controls.

(Schreiber et al., 1994). Adult male Fisher rats were sacrificed either one or 3 d after ADX, whereas separate groups received daily injections of corticosterone (CORT) postoperatively. Three days after ADX, increased p53 gene expression was observed only in those granule cells exhibiting morphological features of apoptosis (Fig. 3). Daily CORT replacement for 3 d significantly attenuated both p53 induction and granule cell death (Fig. 3), suggesting that CORT negatively regulates p53 transcription. The pattern of cells with DNA fragmentation closely paralleled that of p53 induction (Fig. 1E), and DNA damage was prevented by CORT replacement. Under higher magnification, fragmented chromatin could be visualized within apoptotic cells (Fig. 1F). Taken together, the results of these investigations confirm that the relationship between DNA damage, p53 induction, and apoptosis described previously can also be applied to the CNS. Thus, in two distinct models of neuronal apoptosis a clear correlation between the regional distribution and cellular specificity of increased p53 mRNA expression and DNA fragmentation was evident. Further, comparison of the temporal profiles of p53 induction and DNA fragmentation in vitro (Fig. 2) implies that p53 may contribute to the activation of endonucleases proposed to be responsible for oligonucleosomal DNA cleavage. Colocalization of p53 induction and DNA fragmentation not only provides strong support for p53 as a marker of neuronal apoptosis, but also suggests an active role for p53 in the neuronal death process. Since the p53 protein is an important cell cycle regulator that mediates its function primarily through transcriptional regulation, it follows that other p53-inducible, cell cycle-related genes might be involved. Additional work will be necessary to determine whether p53 expression is required for neuronal apoptosis, and if genes, such as waf1 are also upregulated.

6. Other Evidence Linking p53 and Neuronal Death

Recent studies have provided supportive evidence for a relationship between p53 gene activation and neuronal death in the CNS. Following middle cerebral artery occlusion, increased p53 mRNA and protein were detected in regions of severe neuronal damage, but were not localized to specific cell types (Li et al., 1994). Similar results have been obtained following photochemical brain injury (Manev et al., 1994). Thus, p53 induction may be a response to a variety of insults that result in permanent neuronal loss. The availability of transgenic mice expressing a p53 null allele will enable the role of p53 to be more precisely defined (Donehower et al., 1992). Using these mice, Crumrine et al. (1994) have shown that loss of p53 affords relative protection against focal ischemic neuronal damage. In addition, cerebellar granule cells in p53 null mice are resistant to radiation-induced apoptosis (Wood and Youle, 1995). However, p53 knockout mice exhibit a normal phenotype indicating that spontaneous neuronal death during early development is p53-independent. Nonetheless, the evidence described here supports the premise that p53-dependent apoptosis occurs in the CNS, and could be important in the pathophysiology of selective neuronal vulnerability. In this regard, Alzheimer's and Huntington's diseases, as well as other disorders characterized by the loss of specific neuronal populations may be associated with increased p53 expression. Whether the p53 protein is a so-called "killer protein" that could be a potential target of pharmacologic modalities remains to be determined.

Summary

The p53 tumor suppressor gene encodes a cell cycle regulator that has also been implicated in apoptosis. Studies were undertaken to investigate the role of p53 in two different models of neuronal apoptosis in the CNS. Following either systemic KA treatment or adrenalectomy, apoptotic neurons expressed increased p53 mRNA. *In situ* labeling revealed fragmented DNA in apoptotic neurons; the distribution of cells containing fragmented DNA was similar to that of p53 induction. Similar findings were observed in organotypic hippocampal cultures treated with either KA or NMDA. These results indicate that p53 induction is a marker of neuronal apoptosis and suggest that the p53 protein is actively involved in the death pathway.

References

Cohen J. J. (1993) Apoptosis. *Immunol. Today* **14,** 126–130.

Colotta F., Polentarutti N., Sironi M., and Mantovani A. (1992) Expression and involvement of c-fos and c-jun protooncogenes in programmed cell death induced by growth factor deprivation in lymphoid cell lines. *J. Biol. Chem.* **267,** 18,278–18,283.

Crumrine R. C., Thomas A. L., and Morgan P. F. (1994) Attenuation of p53 expression protects against focal ischemic damage in transgenic mice. *J. Cereb. Blood Flow Metab.* **14,** 887–891.

Donehower L. A., Harvey M., Slagle B. L., McArthur M. J., Montgomery C. A. Jr., Butel J. S., and Bradley A. (1992) Mice deficient for p53 are developmentally normal but susceptible to spontaneous tumours. *Nature* **356,** 215–221.

Dragunow M., Beilharz E., Sirimanne E., Lawlor p., Williams C., Bravo R., and Gluckman P. (1994) Immediate-early gene protein expression in neurons undergoing delayed death but not necrosis following hypoxic-ischemic injury to the young rat brain. *Mol. Brain Res.* **25**, 19–33.

El-Deiry W. S., Harper J. W., O'Connor P. M., Velculescu V. E., Canman C. E., Jackman J., Pietenpol J. A., Burrell M., Hill D. E., Wang Y., Wiman K. G., Mercer W. E., Kastan M. B., Kohn K. W., Elledge S. J., Kinzler K. W., and Vogelstein B. (1994) WAF1/CIP1 is induced in p53-mediated G1 arrest and apoptosis. *Cancer Res.* **54**, 1169–1174.

Farmer G., Bargonetti J., Zhu H., Friedman P., Prywes R., and Prives C. (1992) Wild-type p53 activates transcription in vitro. *Nature* **358**, 83–86.

Filipowski R. K., Hetman M., Kaminska B., and Kaczmarek L. (1994) DNA fragmentation in rat brain after intraperitoneal administration of kainate. *NeuroReport* **5**, 1538–1540.

Freeman R. S., Estus S., and Johnson E. M. (1994) Analysis of cell cycle-related gene expression in postmitotic neurons: selective induction of cyclin D1 during programmed cell death. *Neuron* **12**, 343–355.

Ham J., Babij C., Whitfield J., Pfarr C. M., Lallemand D., Yaniv M., and Rubin L. L. (1995) A c-Jun dominant negative mutant protects sympathetic neurons against programmed cell death. *Neuron* **14**, 927–939.

Heron A., Pollard H., Dessi F., Moreau J., Lasbennes F., Ben-Ari Y., and Charriaut-Marlangue C. (1993) Regional variability in DNA fragmentation after global ischemia evidenced by combined histological and gel electrophoresis observations in the rat brain. *J. Neurochem.* **61**, 1973–1976.

Hollstein M., Sidransky D., Vogelstein B., and Harris C. C. (1991) p53 mutations in human cancers. *Science* **253**, 49–53.

Kastan M. B., Onyerkwere O., Sidransky D., Vogelstein B., and Craig R. W. (1991) Participation of p53 protein in the cellular response to DNA damage. *Cancer Res.* **53**, 6304–6311.

Kern S. E., Kinzler K. W., Bruskin A., Jarosz D., Friedman P., Prives C., and Vogelstein B. (1991) Identification of p53 as a sequence-specific DNA-binding protein. *Science* **252**, 1708–1711.

Kuerbitz S. J., Plunkett B. S., Walsh W. V., and Kastan M. B. (1992) Wild-type p53 is a cell cycle checkpoint determinant following irradiation. *Proc. Natl. Acad. Sci. USA* **89**, 7491–7495.

Lane D. P. (1992) p53, guardian of the genome. *Nature* **358**, 15,16.

Lassman H., Bancher C., Breitschopf H., Wegiel J., Bobinski M., Jellinger K., and Wisniewski H. M. (1995) Cell death in Alzheimer's disease evaluated by DNA fragmentation *in situ. Acta Neuropathol.* **89**, 35–41.

Levine A. J., Momand J., and Finlay C. A. (1991) The p53 tumor suppressor gene. *Nature* **351**, 453–456.

Li Y., Chopp M., Zhang Z. G., Zaloga C., Niewenhuis L., and Gautam S. (1994) p53-immunoreactive protein and p53 mRNA expression after transient middle cerebral artery occlusion in rats. *Stroke* **25,** 849–856.

MacManus J. P., Hill I. E., Huang Z.-G., Rasquinha I., Xue D., and Buchan A. M. (1994) DNA damage consistent with apoptosis in transient focal ischaemic neocortex. *NeuroReport* **5,** 493–496.

Manev H., Kharlamov A., and Armstrong D. M. (1994) Photochemical brain injury in rats triggers DNA fragmentation p53 and HSP72. *NeuroReport* **5,** 2661–2664.

Nitecka L., Tremblay E., Charton G., Bouillot J. P., Berger M. L., and Ben-Ari Y. (1984) Maturation of kainic acid seizure-brain damage syndrome in the rat. II. Histo-pathological sequelae. *Neuroscience* **13,** 1073–1094.

Pollard H., Charriaut-Marlangue C., Cantagrel S., Represa A., Robain O., Moreau J., and Ben-Ari Y. (1994) Kainate-induced apoptotic cell death in hippocampal neurons. *Neuroscience* **63,** 7–18.

Portera-Cailliau C., Hedreen J. C., Price D. L., and Koliatsos V. E. (1995) Evidence for apoptotic cell death in Huntington disease and excitotoxic animal models. *J. Neurosci.* **15,** 3775–3787.

Ryan J. J., Danish R., Gottlieb C. A., and Clarke M. F. (1993) Cell cycle analysis of p53-induced death in murine erythroleukemia cells. *Mol. Cell Biol.* **13,** 711–719.

Sakhi S., Bruce A., Sun N., Tocco G., Baudry M., and Schreiber S. S. (1994) p53 induction is associated with neuronal damage in the central nervous system. *Proc. Natl. Acad. Sci. USA* **91,** 7525–7529.

Sakhi S., Bruce A., Sun N., Tocco G., Baudry M., and Schreiber S. S. (1995) Excitotoxin-induced apoptosis in organotypic hippocampal cultures: p53 upregulation and DNA fragmentation. *Exp. Neurol.,* in press.

Schreiber S. S., Sakhi S., Millicent M. Dugich-Djordjevic and Nichols N. R. (1994) Tumor suppressor p53 induction and DNA damage in hippocampal granule cells after adrenalectomy. *Exp. Neurol.* **130,** 368–376.

Schreiber S. S., Tocco G., Najm I., Thompson R. F., and Baudry M. (1993) Cycloheximide prevents kainate-induced neuronal death and c-fos expression in adult rat brain *J. Mol. Neurosci.* **4,** 149–159.

Schwob J. E., Fuller T., Price J. L., and Olney J. W. (1980) Widespread patterns of neuronal damage following systemic or intracerebral injections of kainic acid: a histological study. *Neuroscience* **5,** 991–1014.

Shaw P., Bovey R., Tardy S., Sahli R., Sordat B., and Costa J. (1992) Induction of apoptosis by wild-type p53 in a human colon tumor-derived cell line. *Proc. Natl. Acad. Sci. USA* **89,** 4495–4499.

Shi Y., Glynn J. M., Guilbert L. J., Cotter T. G., Bissonnette R. P., and Green D. R. (1992) Role for c-myc in activation-induced apoptotic cell death in T cell hybridomas. *Science* **257,** 212–214.

Sloviter R. S., Dean E., and Neubort S. (1993a) Electron microscopic analysis of adrenalectomy-induced hippocampal granule cell degeneration in the rat: apoptosis in the adult central nervous system. *J. Comp. Neurol.* **330,** 337–351.

Sloviter R. S., Sollas A. L., Dean E., and Neubort S. (1993b) Adrenalectomy-induced granule cell degeneration in the rat hippocampal dentate gyrus: characterization of an in vivo model of controlled neuronal death *J. Comp. Neurol.* **330,** 324–336.

Smeyne R. J., Vendrell M., Hayward M., Baker S. J., Miao G. G., Schilling K., Robertson L. M., Curran T., and Morgan J. I. (1993) Continuous c-fos expression precedes programmed cell death in vivo. *Nature* **363,** 166–169.

Steller H. (1995) Mechanisms and genes of cellular suicide. *Science* **267,** 1445–1449.

Su J. H., Anderson A. J., Cummings B. J., and Cotman C. W. (1994) Immunohistochemical evidence for apoptosis in Alzheimer's disease. *NeuroReport* **5,** 2529–2533.

Thompson C. B. (1995) Apoptosis in the pathogenesis and treatment of disease. *Science* **267,** 1456–1462.

Wood K. A. and Youle R. J. (1995) The role of free radicals and p53 in neuron apoptosis in vivo. *J. Neurosci.* **15,** 5851–5857.

Yonish-Rouach E., Resnitzky D., Lotem J., Sachs L., Kimchi A., and Oren M. (1991) Wild-type p53 induces apoptosis of myeloid leukaemic cells that is inhibited by interleukin-6. *Nature* **352,** 345–347.

Zhan Q., Carrier F., and Fornace A. J., Jr. (1993) Induction of cellular p53 activity by DNA-damaging agents and growth arrest. *Mol. Cell Biol.* **13,** 4242–4250.

Apoptosis and Ischemia in the Central Nervous System

Matthew D. Linnik

1. Introduction

Our understanding of apoptosis and programmed cell death has rapidly evolved over the last decade. As originally conceived, apoptosis was a purely morphological phenomena based on the appearance of membrane blebbing (apoptotic bodies) and nuclear changes, including chromatin condensation and DNA fragmentation. Likewise, programmed cell death was a developmental definition describing the physiologically appropriate "programmed" death of cells during developmental modeling and morphogenesis.

Given these strict definitions, one could exclude programmed cell death in stroke as ischemia-induced cell death is clearly not a normally programmed event. One might also exclude the term apoptosis, as the original papers describing apoptosis specifically cited ischemia as a mechanism to induce coagulative necrotic cell death, as opposed to apoptosis.

Then how might one justify a chapter discussing the methodology associated with apoptosis in stroke? The answer is largely based on the imposition of cellular and molecular biology on the fields of apoptosis and programmed cell death. Whereas the original definitions relied heavily on morphology and cell counting, advances in cellular and molecular biology have led to an expanded definition of apoptosis based on the activation and function of specific genes and gene products. In addition, the ability to model the

From: *Neuromethods, Vol. 29: Apoptosis Techniques and Protocols*
Ed: J. Poirier Humana Press Inc.

developmental programmed cell death of neurons in culture has revealed additional phenomena that can be evaluated in the ischemic brain.

The terminology associated with apoptotic or programmed cell death has triggered much debate (Alles et al., 1991). In this chapter, the term apoptosis will be used to identify the active, intracellular, suicide-like processes that contribute to ischemia-induced death in neurons. It is not meant to imply that the majority of neurons exhibit overt apoptotic morphology after a stroke, although this morphology has recently been reported (Li et al., 1995b, 1995c; Nitatori et al., 1995). Rather, this chapter will identify the data suggesting that apoptotic-like processes occur in stroke and will stress the methodological considerations necessary to build on these investigations.

2. Experimental Stroke Models for Investigating Apoptosis

Several experimental models are available for studying apoptosis in stroke. These can be divided into three major classes, global ischemia, focal ischemia, and thromboembolic models. The methodology and pathophysiology associated with these models have been extensively reviewed (Pulsinelli, 1992; Hsu, 1993; Hossmann, 1994; Hunter et al., 1995) and will be discussed here primarily in the context of apoptosis-related cell death models.

The global ischemia models temporarily restrict cerebral blood flow to the brain in a manner analogous to what might occur during a myocardial infarction. The desired effect is a delayed cell death in a select group of neurons confined to the CA1 region of the hippocampus (Kirino, 1982). The selected vulnerability of the CA1 neurons is exclusive to the hippocampus as virtually all other neurons in the brain are spared.

In contrast to the global models, focal ischemia models restrict blood flow to selected regions of the brain. The majority of focal models restrict blood supply to one of the middle cerebral arteries, resulting in a unilateral infarct confined to the ipsilateral cerebral hemisphere. The volume of infarcted cortical tissue, and the potential involvement of subcortical tissue, is dependent on the location of the occlusion. Proximal occlusions at the origin of the middle cerebral artery produce the largest cortical infarcts and often involve subcortical structures. More distal occlusions cause progressively smaller cortical infarcts with little or no subcortical involvement. The focal models represent the majority of clinical stroke presentations since 60–70% of all strokes are occlusive and the majority of occlusive strokes involve the carotid territory (Sacco, 1994; Kothari et al., 1995)

The thromboembolic models involve the generation of localized intravascular coagulation by exposing a select area of the brain to an appropriate light source after the IV administration of the radical generating dye rose bengal (Watson et al., 1985). Although these models are less frequently used to study ischemic cell death, they offer a unique mechanism to produce ischemia. The infarcted areas produced in the thromboembolic models share many of the pathophysiological features observed in focal ischemia models and exhibit several features consistent with apoptotic cell death (Manev et al., 1994). Thus, whereas the thromboembolic models offer a highly differentiated approach to the generation of ischemia, many of the experimental principals needed to investigate ischemic apoptosis are similar to the focal models and will not be discussed here as an independent subject.

2.1. Global Ischemia and Apoptosis

The rodent global ischemia models originally described by Pulsinelli et al. (1979, 1982) and Kirino et al. (1982) have been carefully studied because of the very selective nature of the cell death that accompanies the ischemia. With brief global ischemia, the cell death occurs in a select group of neurons in the CA1 region of the hippocampus. Remarkably, the death of these neurons is delayed by two or more days, suggesting that brief ischemia initiates a process that requires several hours to days develop.

Global ischemia can be surgically induced by occluding the common carotid arteries and/or vertebral arteries, or, less commonly, by stopping the heart (Mossakowski et al., 1986; Krajewski et al., 1995). The death of CA1 neurons occurs when cerebral blood flow is sufficiently compromised for 5–15 min, a duration that is sufficient to produce an infarct without compromising the ability of the animal to regain consciousness.

In order to assess the mechanisms that contribute to neuronal death in experimental stroke models, one can compare these stroke models with highly characterized models of developmental programmed cell death. The most fully characterized neuronal model is the programmed cell death of superior cervical ganglia cultures that have been deprived of nerve growth factor (NGF) (Martin et al., 1988). In this model, NGF removal from cultured ganglia neurons causes a delayed neuronal death that exhibits several features of apoptosis, including dependence on macromolecular synthesis, nucleosomal DNA fragmentation, protection by anti-apoptotic proteins like bcl-2, and an irreversible commitment to cell death between 18 and 24 h after removal of the NGF (Martin et al., 1988, 1992; Deckworth and Johnson, 1993).

The comparison between hippocampal cell death in the global ischemia model and the death of superior cervical ganglia neurons after NGF removal is striking. First, the neurons in both models become committed to die before they exhibit any morphological evidence of injury. Second, both models exhibit DNA fragmentation into nucleosomal ladders. Third, the death of neurons can be prevented by supplementation with NGF if added before the cells are committed to die (Shigeno et al., 1991; Yamamoto et al., 1992; Pechan et al., 1995). Finally, the neuronal death in both models can be prevented by inhibiting new protein synthesis (Martin et al., 1988; Papas et al., 1992).

Whereas many features of the global ischemia models are desirable, these models pose technical challenges for studying apoptotic phenomena in vivo. The limited tissue volume of CA1 neurons and the bilateral nature of the damage make quantitative biochemical and molecular studies difficult. The quantitation of cell death in the hippocampus is also labor intensive, as damage is assessed by counting individual cells or by scoring damage on a predetermined scale. Finally, it has been reported that the CA1 neurons do not exhibit apoptotic morphology as there is an absence of chromatin condensation or apoptotic bodies preceding frank neuronal degeneration (Deshpande et al., 1992). However, other investigators have suggested the possibility of apoptotic physiology and morphology in partial global ischemia (Islam et al., 1995; Nitatori et al., 1995).

2.2. Focal Ischemia and Apoptosis

Focal cerebral ischemia can be generated in animals by procedures that invade the intracranial space or by other relatively noninvasive procedures. In the invasive models, a craniotomy is performed to visualize the middle cerebral artery prior to occlusion. In noninvasive models, a monofilament is advanced from the internal carotid artery in the neck to the occlude middle cerebral artery without opening the scull. Both models can be used to produce permanent or transient ischemia and several variations of these models have been described.

The focal ischemia models exhibit many of the biochemical and molecular features that suggest a process resembling apoptosis is occurring. These include features related to DNA fragmentation, dependence on macromolecular synthesis, appearance and functional role for apoptosis-specific proteins, and evidence for apoptotic morphology (Shigeno et al., 1990; Heron et al., 1993; Linnik et al., 1993b, 1995b; MacManus et al., 1994; Li et al., 1995a,b,c; Krajewski et al., 1995). These observations and others will be discussed in greater detail in later sections.

The focal models have been very instructive as they have a predictable time course and allow one to generate sufficient tissue for biochemical and molecular investigations. Furthermore, the focal models mimic the most prevalent human strokes and observations in these models may have an immediate applicability to human pathophysiology.

The focal ischemia models produce infarctions in contiguous groups of cells. This conflicts with early definitions of apoptosis suggesting that necrosis affects tracts of cells, whereas apoptosis affects select cells in a given tissue. However, there are now several examples, in which large, continuous group of cells die by genetically programmed cell death, including the intercostal muscles of *Manduca sexta* (Schwartz et al., 1993) and the developing nervous system (Oppenheim, 1991).

2.3. General Considerations Related to Stroke Models

There are two important caveats to bear in mind as one contemplates cell death experiments in stroke models. First, the stroke models must be conducted under extremely well controlled conditions. Stroke models are notoriously sensitive to a number of physiological variables, including core temperature, blood glucose, and blood pCO_2 levels. Alterations in these variables can dramatically alter the pathological outcome, and these factors must be controlled to allow for clear interpretation of data. Excellent discussions on the effect of temperature (Buchan and Pulsinelli, 1990; Ginsberg et al., 1992), blood glucose (Yip et al., 1991), and CO_2 (Tulleken and Abraham, 1975) are available.

The second caveat is the understanding that some degree of necrosis also contributes to cell death in focal ischemia models (MacManus et al., 1995). The necrotic death is most evident in the core of the infarction in which the reduction in cerebral blood flow is so severe that the primary cause of death is energy failure (Li et al., 1995d; Linnik et al., 1995b). To further complicate matters, apoptotic death can assume a necrotic morphology in terminal stages (Wyllie et al., 1980). Because of the selective vulnerability of different neurons to ischemia, the death of neurons after a stroke is not synchronous, and cells that originally appear apoptotic can proceed to necrosis. Thus, observations in stroke models may include a combination of necrosis and apoptosis, and the criteria for deciding exactly where necrosis stops and apoptosis starts are more difficult to interpret in nonconcentric, postmitotitic cells like neurons.

Finally, it is generally accepted that consultation with an experienced investigator will facilitate the implementation of any new model. This principal is especially true for stroke models. If you are considering implementing one or more stroke models for experimental analysis, one should strongly consider visiting an established laboratory as it will almost certainly save many hours during the implementation and validation of the model.

3. Apoptotic Morphology in Stroke

The subject of apoptotic morphology has been among the more controversial aspects of studying apoptosis in stroke. The original definition of apoptosis was based on morphology and included the following criteria: chromatin condensation and margination to the nuclear membrane, cell shrinkage with marked crowding of organelles, and membrane blebbing to form apoptotic bodies (Kerr et al., 1972; Wyllie et al., 1980). In addition, all events occur in absence of lymphocyte infiltration or exudative inflammation. Notable in these descriptions was the specific citation of ischemia as a mechanism to produce coagulative necrosis (Kerr et al., 1972; Wyllie et al., 1980).

The question of whether a biochemical apoptosis or programmed death could occur in the absence of apoptotic morphology was addressed by Schwartz and colleagues (1993). These investigators compared the programmed cell death of the interstitial muscles in the moth, *Manduca sexta*, with the apoptotic death of thymocytes exposed to glucocorticoids. These two well-described models of active cell death displayed differences in cell surface morphology, nuclear ultrastructure, and DNA fragmentation, suggesting the existence of tissue-specific morphology in physiologically programmed cell deaths.

The morphology of neurons during ischemic cell death have been evaluated in global and focal models with surprising results. The delayed neuronal death observed in global ischemia initially suggested an excellent opportunity to evaluate the possibility of apoptotic morphology in stroke. Deshpande et al. (1992) reported a detailed study in which they used light and electron microscopy to look for evidence of apoptosis in CA1 hippocampal neurons after 10 min of global ischemia. They observed that the most prominent early feature of delayed neuronal death was polysome disggregation, and that the mitochondrial and nuclear elements remained intact until frank neuronal degeneration. The authors concluded that delayed neuronal death does not exhibit the prominent features of apoptosis.

In contrast, Nitatori et al. (1995) recently examined delayed neuronal death in the CA1 pyramidal cell layer using light and electron microscopy, as well as extensive lysosomal proteinase histochemistry. These investigators reported that the mitochondria are intact when nuclear changes initiate and concluded that this cell death exhibits apoptotic morphology. Thus, the issue of whether apoptotic morphology occurs in global ischemia remains controversial.

The focal ischemia models produce a more rapid death that involves a large contiguous tract of cells and likely contains a core of frank necrotic cell death. Using light and electron microscopy methods, Li et al. (1995a,b,c) demonstrated isolated neurons that exhibited several classic features of apoptosis including chromatin aggregation, cytoplasmic condensation, and the appearance of apoptotic bodies containing fragments of condensed nuclear chromatin.

Thus, the currently available data suggests that apoptotic morphology can be demonstrated in focal ischemia, whereas the conclusions regarding global ischemia are more controversial. For those wishing to extend these observations, the methodology involves standard light and electron microscopy techniques. The references that best distinguish apoptosis from necrosis include the original reports (Kerr et al., 1972, 1995; Wyllie et al., 1980). In applying this technology to ischemia, one should recognize that apoptotic cell deaths can degenerate into necrotic morphology. Thus, it is prudent to evaluate the tissue at several time points after the ischemia to get a clear picture of the progression of the cell death.

4. DNA Fragmentation in Stroke

One of the hallmarks of apoptosis is the early and rapid digestion of the nuclear DNA by endonucleases. Several laboratories have now demonstrated apoptotic DNA fragmentation in the brain after focal and global ischemia (Heron et al., 1993; Linnik et al., 1993b, 1995b; Okamoto et al., 1993; MacManus et al., 1993, 1994; Tominaga et al., 1993; Li et al., 1995a,b). DNA fragmentation can be observed as soon as 0.5–4 h after initiation of focal cerebral ischemia and 12–24 h after global ischemia. The onset of DNA fragmentation is early in the cell death process since no morphological evidence of cell death is apparent at this time.

In focal ischemia, the DNA fragmentation appears to be concentrated around the inner boundary zone of the infarction rather than in the core of the infarction where necrosis might be expected to predominate (Li et al., 1995a,b; Linnik et al., 1995b). The boundary zone tissue is also the tissue that is amenable to pharmacologic intervention in experimental studies. Thus, it appears that apoptosis concentrates in the salvageable tissue of the penumbra, whereas necrosis predominates in areas where the sustained lack of blood flow may make tissue salvage impossible.

4.1. Gel Electrophoresis for Oligonucleosomal Fragmentation

As cells die, the DNA can be digested in a specific fashion by endonucleases, suggesting apoptosis, or in a random manner by lysosomal enzymes, suggesting necrosis (MacManus et al., 1995). When the DNA is size-fractionated by gel electrophoresis, endonucleolytic digestion results in the classical oligonucleosomal ladder pattern, whereas lysosomal cleavage yields a smear of DNA. The oligonucleosomal ladders are thought to result from the specific cleavage of DNA by endonucleases at the accessible internucleosomal regions. Since focal ischemia models exhibit a combination of necrosis (primarily at the core of the lesion) and apoptosis (primarily arising from the perimeter of the lesion), the DNA extracted from an ischemic cortex can be expected to exhibit oligonucleosomal ladders on a background of randomly degraded DNA.

The basic methods for analyzing the integrity of DNA involve the following steps: homogenization of the tissues or cells in detergent, removal of protein and RNA by enzymatic digestion and phenol extraction, DNA concentration by precipitation in ethanol, size fractionation by agarose gel electrophoresis, and visualization of the DNA by ethidium bromide staining or radiolabeling procedures.

It has been our observation that oligonucleosomal fragments can be more easily visualized if the low-mol wt DNA is separated from the high-mol wt chromatin immediately after the initial homogenization. This can be accomplished by a simple centrifugation of the original homogenate, provided the tissue has not been previously treated with proteinase K. This partial purification also has the added advantage of making the DNA easier to manipulate in subsequent steps since the viscous, high-mol wt DNA will have been removed.

4.1.1. Oligonucleosomal DNA Extraction Procedure

1. Rapidly remove brain into ice-cold PBS, dissect region of interest, place in lysis buffer (20 m*M* Tris, pH 7.4, 10 m*M* EDTA, 0.1% Triton X-100), and mince with scissors on ice. Incubate for 20–30 min with intermittent trituration to facilitate lysis.

2. Centrifuge homogenate at 13,000*g* for 20 min to separate low molecular weight DNA from the high molecular weight chromatin in the pellet. The high-mol wt chromatin pellet is small, clear, and difficult to visualize until the desired supernatant is removed. Also, note that the high molecular weight DNA will not pellet if the chromatin structure has been disrupted by prior protease treatment.

3. Collect supernatant and digest with 100 μg/mL proteinase K and 100 μg/mL DNase-free RNase A for 2 h at 37°C.

4. Remove protein by adding an equal volume of Tris saturated phenol:chloroform:isoamyl alcohol (25:24:1) to the samples, gently vortex, and centrifuge in a microcentrifuge at full speed (approx 13,000g) for 5 min.
5. Collect supernatant without disturbing the interface and re-extract with chloroform:isoamyl alcohol (24:1) using same centrifugation conditions.
6. Collect supernatant and precipitate DNA in ethanol (30 µL 3M NaAc, 0.5 µL 0.5M MgCl$_2$-6H$_2$O, then 1000 µL 100% EtOH for a 300-µL sample) at –70°C for > 6 h. The magnesium chloride is added to enhance the recovery of the small DNA fragments.
7. Pellet DNA for 30 min at 4°C in microcentrifuge, remove EtOH, gently rinse pellet with 80% ethanol, aspirate EtOH, and dry briefly at room temperature or in a vacuum concentrator.
8. Rehydrate DNA in 20 µL water, add 3 µL loading buffer and electrophorese at 30 mA overnight in a 1.8% agarose gel containing ethidium bromide in 1X TBE. Alternatively, run the gel at 50 mA approx 3–6 h. Visualize the bands by exposing the gel to a UV light source.

If the tissue source is limited, as in the hippocampus, the recovery of fragmented DNA may be too limited to visualize by standard ethidium bromide staining. In these cases, the DNA signal can be amplified by labeling the DNA with radioactive nucleotides prior to gel electrophoresis. When using this procedure, it is preferable to collect total DNA to minimize any losses of low-mol wt DNA that could occur during purification. The following procedure has been used successfully to demonstrate and quantitate the extent of DNA fragmentation (Sei et al., 1994; MacManus et al., 1994).

4.1.2. Radiolabeling Oligonucleosomal DNA Fragments

1. Incubate 10 µg of DNA with 15 µCi of [α^{32}P]-dideoxyATP (3000 Ci/mmol) and 15 U of terminal transferase in 50 µL of 0.1 mM potassium cacodylate, 2 mM CoCl, and 0.2 mM dithiothreitol at pH 7.2 for 30 min.

2. Stop the reaction by the addition of 2 μL of 0.5 mM EDTA.
3. Precipitate the DNA in ethanol (*see* Section 4.1.1., steps 6–7).
4. Separate the DNA by electrophoresis in a 1.8% agarose gel at 40 mA until the bands in the marker ladders can be discriminated. A good marker ladder for these gels is the 123-bp ladder (Gibco-BRL, Gaithersburg, MD).
5. Carefully remove the gel, wrap in plastic wrap, and visualize the DNA by exposing the gel to film or phosphoimager screen for several hours to days.

The above procedure has the added advantage that the each lane can be sliced out of the gel and counted for radioactivity, thus providing a means of directly quantitating the results.

4.2. Initial Endonuclease Activation

Most methods for evaluating the DNA digestion in apoptosis concentrate on oligonucleosome fragments <10,000 bp. These observations may be unnecessarily biased toward small fragments since the initial destruction of the genome into larger fragments is sufficient to cause the chromatin condensation characteristic of apoptosis (Walker et al., 1994). Recent observations suggest that the initial activation of endonucleases in apoptosis leads to a multiphasic destruction of the genome that begins with the appearance of very large DNA fragments. In thymocytes, hepatocytes, and PC12 cells, the DNA was shown to fragment into 300-kb bands that subsequently degraded in a stepwise fashion to 50-kb bands before exhibiting smaller oligonucleosome fragments (Walker et al., 1993, 1994; Pandey et al., 1994). In addition, it is possible that unique endonucleases are responsible for internucleosomal and high molecular mass DNA fragmentation during apoptosis (Pandey et al., 1994).

Recent studies suggest that the DNA degradation in reversible focal ischemia also proceeds in this stepwise fashion. Using pulsed field methodology, Charriaut-Marlangue et al. (1995) demonstrated the degradation of cerebral cortex DNA into 300-kb fragments, followed by further digestion to 50-kb fragments, and finally smaller oligonucleosomal fragments. The 300-kb fragments were maximal at 6 h post-ischemia (the first time point measured) and were declining by 18 h as the smaller fragments began to predominate.

Special methods are required to handle large DNA fragments to prevent spurious DNA breaks occurring as a consequence of handling the material. Typically, cells are embedded in agarose plugs before proteinase digestion to minimize pipet-induced shearing. Second, the DNA must be electrophoresed in a nonlinear manner to allow the large strands to separate from each other. This can be accomplished by either pulsed field or field inversion gel electrophoresis. In either approach, one should be careful to establish electrophoresis parameters that allow for resolution of the band of interest as one can generate artifactual compression of the DNA by choosing inappropriate electrophoresis parameters. Investigators interested in applying these techniques should refer to the indicated references and the literature provided by the equipment manufacturers.

4.3. In Situ *Labeling of DNA Ends*

Gavrieli et al. (1992) were the first to report a technique for identifying cells with DNA damage in tissue sections. The method is often identified as TUNEL staining, an acronym for terminal deoxynucleotidyl transferase dUTP nick-end labeling. TUNEL staining employs the enzyme terminal transferase, which adds a labeled deoxynucleotide to free 3' hydroxyl ends of DNA. The number of free DNA ends accumulates as the DNA is damaged causing these to cells stain more intensely than normal cells.

The development of procedures that identify DNA fragmentation *in situ* was initially adopted with great enthusiasm. The techniques were readily implemented and began to be used to "identify" apoptotic cell death. It was soon recognized that *in situ* DNA end labeling does not discriminate between apoptotic cell deaths and necrotic cell deaths, and the technique was appropriately criticized. The reality is that TUNEL staining can be very useful for measuring DNA damage, but one must recognize that TUNEL staining cannot be used in isolation to discriminate between apoptotic cells and necrotic cells.

Bearing these caveats in mind, several laboratories have found that the *in situ* DNA end labeling procedures are quite useful for at least two types of observations in stroke. First, they permit one to determine the time course for the development of DNA degradation after a stroke. In focal ischemia models, the initial appearance of DNA degradation was observed as early as 0.5 h (Li et al., 1995b) to 1 h (Linnik et al., 1995) after middle cerebral artery occlusion. In global ischemia, the DNA fragmentation in the CA1 neurons has been reported as early as 12 h after ischemia (Sei et al., 1994), whereas others report variable fragmentation beginning at 24 h (Heron et al., 1993; MacManus et al., 1995).

These above mentioned studies have important implications related to the mechanisms of cell death after a stroke. In the focal models, histological evidence of cellular damage is not apparent for 4–6 h after ischemia. Likewise, in global ischemia models, histological evidence of cellular damage is not apparent for 48 h after ischemia (Kirino, 1982; Pulsinelli et al., 1982). Thus, in both focal and global ischemia, the appearance of DNA damage is a very early event in the cell death cycle and precedes the morphological appearance of tissue damage.

The DNA labeling procedures have also contributed to determining the length of ischemia necessary for subsequent cell death. Li et al. (1995b) showed that the number of cells with DNA fragmentation increases with prolonged ischemia, beginning with occlusions as short as 10 min. In a different focal model, MacManus et al. (1994) also reported an increase in the number of TUNEL-positive cells as the duration of ischemia was increased.

The second area where the *in situ* DNA labeling techniques have been useful is determining the regional localization of DNA fragmentation in the brain after a stroke. For example, Li et al. (1995d) used TUNEL staining to demonstrate that DNA fragmentation concentrates along the inner boundary zone of the infarction. This area is often referred to as the penumbra and is the area where pharmacologic interventions are capable of rescuing tissue from ischemic damage. The TUNEL staining has been particularly useful in global ischemia, where one is evaluating the selective cell death in the hippocampal cells in the CA1 region (MacManus et al., 1993).

It should be reemphasized that TUNEL staining procedures do not differentiate between necrosis and apoptosis. However, they can serve as one of several observations that form the basis of discriminating between apoptosis and necrosis. At a minimum, one should consider supporting a positive TUNEL result with evidence that an endonuclease is responsible for the observed DNA damage.

The techniques for TUNEL staining are well described and will not be reproduced here. We have employed the original method of Gavrieli et al. (1992) as well as the commercially available ApopTag kit (Oncor, Gaithersburg, MD). The Gavrieli method adds biotinylated dUTP to the free 3' OH of the DNA and develops the biotin with Extra-avidin peroxidase. In the Oncor method, the DNA ends are labeled with dUTP. An antidigoxigenein antibody coupled to peroxidase is bound to the digoxigenin and color is generated by addition of a peroxidase-sensitive chromogenic substrate. In our experience, either method can be used to provide acceptable results. In practice, we have observed that the catalytic action of the peroxidase in the Oncor method provides a greater differential between normal cells and apoptotic cells in the same section. This differential may facilitate the identification of positive cells when employing an automated image analyzer for quantitating the number of apoptotic cells in a section.

4.4. Analyzing Neurons by Flow Cytometry

The flow cytometer is designed for quantitative, multiparametric analyses of isolated cells and has been used extensively for the characterization of apoptosis in lymphocytes (Darzynkiewicz et al., 1992; Dive et al., 1992). In contrast, flow cytometry has received little exposure in the nervous system due to the substrate dependent nature of neurons and the structural limitations associated with the axonal and dendritic arbor.

The flow cytometer aligns cells in a stream and analyzes each cell individually by passing the cell through a laser beam of fixed wavelength. A fluorometric detection system permits analysis of absorbance, transmission, or specific wavelength emission. The number of parameters that can be determined for any individual cell is limited by the nature of the signals and the sophistication of the detection system. In practice, one can readily analyze 2–3 surface markers and obtain a DNA profile on each of 30,000–50,000 cells in a single sample analysis. The data can then be plotted as a population distribution to determine if there is correlation between any of the parameters that were measured.

The primary limitation for analysis of neurons in the flow cytometer is that the instrument requires isolated cells that are free of debris. This is the normal state for lymphocytes, but is more difficult to accomplish with substrate dependent, nonconcentric neurons. The samples do not have to be absolutely clean, as the flow cytometer can exclude cell fragments and clumps of cells. However, the most accurate signal is obtained when the cells are adequately digested and purified.

We have utilized the flow cytometer to evaluate cell shrinkage and DNA fragmentation in neuroblastoma cells in vitro (Linnik et al., 1993a) and DNA fragmentation in isolated neurons after focal cerebral ischemia (Linnik et al., 1993b, 1995). In this procedure, individual cells are isolated from the ischemic and nonischemic cortex, stained with propidium iodide to identify the DNA, and analyzed using the flow cytometer. It should be emphasized that these methods are not fully optimized and several modifications might be considered depending on the type of investigation. However, this procedure will provide large numbers of relatively discrete, fixed neurons that are amenable to flow cytometric analysis.

The critical components for preparing discrete cell populations from a normal or ischemic brain are the rapid fixation of the brain, rehydration of the brain to make it amenable to enzymatic digestion, and a brief discontinuous density gradient centrifugation to separate the debris (primarily axons and dendrites) from the cell bodies.

4.1.1. Isolating Neurons for Flow Cytometry

1. Deeply anesthetize the animal and perfuse the brain with fixative by opening the chest, exposing the heart, and perfusing the animal with 100 mL of saline followed by 100 mL of 10% formalin in phosphate-buffered saline. Perfusion fixation is essential to preserve the integrity of the DNA. Occasionally animals are identified that do not receive good cranial perfusions and these animals should be excluded from further DNA analysis.

2. Remove the brain, dissect into regions of interest and postfix regions by soaking in 10% formalin in phosphate-buffered saline for 0.5–2 h.

3. Begin the process of removing formaldehyde by soaking the tissue in an excess of 70% EtOH in PBS for 30 min with gentle agitation. The formaldehyde must be removed or it will inactivate the enzymes used to digest the tissue.

4. Remove the remainder of the formaldehyde and the EtOH by rehydrating the tissue through a graded series of EtOH into 100% PBS. We use 50% EtOH for 10 min, 30% EtOH for 10 min, and 3X 100% PBS for 10 min each with gentle agitation on an orbit shaker. Recent observations in lymphocytes suggest that cells can be adequately rehydrated by extensive washing with phosphate-buffered saline (Gibellini et al., 1995). This should eliminate the need for the EtOH rehydration steps, however, we have not fully evaluated the effect of this modification on the neurons.

5. Resuspended the tissue in 5 mL of Earles balanced salt solution (EBSS) with 1X trypsin, mince, and gently triturated with a 10-mL pipet for approx 5 min. The timing for the digestion is determined empirically and is complete when the tissue is ≤ 50% digested and the solution is cloudy. Further digestion will result in extensive cell fragmentation and should be avoided.

6. Add 10% serum to inactivate the trypsin and allow remaining pieces of tissue to settle to the bottom. Collect the supernatant and centrifuge at 300g for 5 min at room temperature to isolate a cell pellet.

7. Prepare a solution of EBSS containing 10 mg/mL ovomucoid inhibitor and 10 mg/mL albumin (EBSS-albumin). Also prepare a dilution of EBSS-albumin containing 2.7 mL of EBSS + 0.3 mL EBSS-albumin. A lyophilized preparation of the ovomucoid albumin mixture is available from Worthington Biochemical (Freehold, NJ).

8. Resuspend the cell pellet from step 6 in 1–3 mL of the diluted EBSS–albumin solution and prepare a discontinuous density gradient by carefully layering the cell suspension on top of 5 mL of EBSS-albumin solution.

9. Centrifuge gradient at 70g for 6 min at room temperature. Dissociated cells will form a loose pellet at the bottom of the tube and membrane fragments will remain in the gradient.

10. Carefully aspirate the supernatant and resuspend the pelleted cells in phosphate-buffered saline at 1×10^6 cells/mL.

11. Incubate cells with 0.5 µg DNase-free RNase for 30 min at 37°C.

12. Place cells on ice and add 50 µg/mL propidium iodide. Vortex gently and incubate in the dark at room temperature for 15 min.

13. Inject sample into flow cytometer for analysis. Using an Elite Flow Cytometer (Coulter Electronics, Hialeah, CA) or similar instrument, collect data on cells emitting at >610 nm on excitation with a 15 mW argon laser.

5. Molecular Approaches to Apoptosis in Stroke

Much of the evidence for neuronal apoptosis in ischemic disorders has been derived from biochemical and molecular studies. In addition, several investigators have sought to adapt information gathered from genetic studies in other experimental models and apply them to the central nervous system. In particular, it has been desirable to determine if the apoptotic genes that are conserved across many species are involved in ischemic cell death.

There are a limited number of technologies that are available for manipulating genes in neurons in vivo. In particular, it has been difficult to establish a selective genetic manipulation in discrete populations of postmitotic neurons. Two systems that have been applied to the investigation of cell death in stroke are viral-based gene expression vectors and transgenic technology. Both methods can be used to gain or delete a specific function by inserting or deleting the gene of interest.

The application of these technologies is in its infancy as it relates to study of apoptosis and ischemic cell death in the central nervous system. In addition, the specific technologies are well beyond the scope of this review. Therefore, this section will concentrate on the methodological parameters that should be considered when applying viral vector technology or transgenic technology to stroke models and experimentation.

5.1. Genetic Manipulation with Viral Vectors

Viral vectors can be used to insert a gene in a specific population of cells. The expression of the gene is accomplished by placing the gene under the control of a promoter sequence that facilitates the assembly of a transcriptional complex at the start of the gene and permits high level transcription of the mRNA of interest. Several different types of promoter elements can be used, including neuron-specific promoters (i.e., neuron-specific enolase promoter) or efficient mammalian or viral promoters.

Two types of viral vectors have been used to increase specific gene expression in stroke, adenoviruses, herpesvirus. Both vectors are capable of delivering genes to postmitotic, terminally differentiated cells. The vectors are typically modifed to reduce or eliminate their ability to replicate autonomously and are identified as replication-deficient vectors. These modifications are necessary to prevent the development of virulent infections and the subsequent complications of uncontrolled virus growth, spread, and localized tissue inflammation and damage. It also provides an enhanced level of safety for the researcher or technician. The modifications that prevent replication of the viruses are not yet foolproof, and in most systems, there is a measurable rate of recombination that permits viral replication. Therefore, extreme caution should be used when working with these viruses in the laboratory.

The viral vectors can be admininstered to the CNS by either direct intraparenchymal injection or injection into the cerebral ventricles. Intraparenchymal injections will favor localized expression in neurons and glial cells, whereas injection into ventricles will favor expression in ependymal cells (Akli et al., 1993; Bajoccchi et al., 1993). Betz et al. (1995) has demonstrated that intracerebroventricular injection of an adenovirus vector expressing human interleukin-1 receptor antagonist protein can attenuate cell death in stroke. In these studies, the expression of protein was confined to cells lining the cerebral ventricles and resulted in 5- to 50-fold increases in interleukin-1β receptor antagonist in the CSF.

The intracerebroventricular injection route is appropriate when one is not concerned about localized increases in expression, but only requires a generalized increase in protein in the circulating CSF. However, for many of the apoptotic specific genes, localized intracellular gene expression is essential. Therefore, a stereotaxic intraparenchymal injection will be the preferred route of administration for many apoptotic genes.

Our laboratory has employed direct intraparenchymal injection of a replication-deficient herpesvirus to evaluate the effect of overexpression of human bcl-2 in stroke (Linnik et al., 1995a). Several methodological considerations were identified that affected the design and execution of these studies, including choice of stroke model, mechanism for injection, and method quantitation and evaluation.

The first consideration was the choice of stroke model. The invasive permanent middle cerebral artery occlusion with tandem ipsilateral common carotid occlusion in the spontaneously hypertensive (SH) rat produces infarctions with a high degree of reproducibility (Chen et al., 1986), and these infarctions are fully developed within 24 h. Because the viral titers that can be injected into the parenchyma are limited, the reproducibility of the SH rat model allows one to accurately predict the location of the infarct and the site for viral vector injection.

The injections require that one use highly concentrated viral titers, as the parenchyma of the brain is relatively intolerant to injection. A concentrated viral stock (1×10^5 infectious particles in 2 µL) can be injected at a rate of 1 µL/4 min using a Hamilton syringe and a Kopf Model 5000 Micro Injection unit (Kopf Instruments, Tujunga, CA). In addition, the needle should be left in the tract for an additional 5 min before retraction to help reduce reflux up the needle tract. There have been reports of investigators injecting up to 10 µL into a site, and our experience would indicate that this would cause a total loss of control over the injection site. Preliminary experimentation with a dye (pontine sky blue) in saline will permit the investigator to gain familiarity with the nature of the injection and the response of the tissue to the injection.

The choice of the vector injection site can be critical, depending on the nature of the observations that are desired. For example, in the case of the HSV-bcl-2 vector, we sought to determine if overexpression of the antiapoptotic gene bcl-2 would provide protection against a subsequent ischemic challenge. To test this hypothesis, overexpression of bcl-2 was required in an area that would be certain to die in the absence of treatment. However, the site of injection had to be outside of the necrotic core to give the vector a reasonable opportunity to exhibit efficacy.

To establish a site of injection, a series of infarcted control animals were analyzed to determine the distance from the midline to the proximal edge of the infarction. This measurement established a lateral coordinate where one could be certain that the injection would be in ischemic tissue. One millimeter lateral was added to account for the necrosis that will be associated with the injection tract. These injection coordinates should be determined empirically for any laboratory.

Establishing the time required for optimal gene expression will facilitate an evaluation of the effect of gene expression on tissue preservation. This is best accomplished using standard immunohistochemistry with an antibody directed against the protein of interest. In the absence of a specific antibody, one can determine mRNA levels by *in situ* hybridization or solution hybridization (RNase protection assay), but these results need to be interpreted cautiously as mRNA expression is not always reflective of actual protein expression.

Several methods can be employed to quantitate the effect of enhanced gene expression on tissue survival in the ischemic brain. The measurement will depend on the route of administration (intracerebroventricular or intraparenchymal) and the nature of the ischemic insult (focal or global ischemia).

5.1.1. Intracerebroventricular Injection and Focal Ischemia

This is the simplest design to implement since one is essentially evaluating the effect of increasing gene expression in the cerebrospinal fluid. In focal ischemia, the brain is removed at 24–72 h after the infarction, sliced into 2-mm saggital sections (six sections per brain), and stained with 2% 2,3,5–triphenyltetrazolium chloride in saline to differentiate live tissue from dead tissue (Park et al., 1988). The dye will stain healthy tissue a bright red, whereas infarcted tissue remains pale white. The volume of the infarction is determined by quantitative video image analysis. It is also possible to estimate edema by comparing the volume of the infarcted hemisphere with the contralateral, normal hemisphere, although our experience suggest that the primary endpoint should be based on infarct volume.

5.1.2. Intracerebroventricular Injection and Global Ischemia

Because global ischemia exclusively targets the CA1 neurons of the hippocampus, there is no overt infarction. Therefore, some method for quantitating individual neuronal loss must be established. The hippocampus can be sectioned, stained with hematoxylin and eosin, and individual cells counted. This method likely produces the most accurate results, but it is tedious and time consuming. An alternative to individual cell counts is an arbitrary scoring system based on relative damage to the CA1 neurons. These methods can be used effectively, provided that the scorers are trained to criteria and are blinded to the control and treatment groups

5.1.3. Intraparenchymal Injection and Focal Ischemia

The small volume of infected cells resulting from intraparenchymal injections requires that quantitation of effect be confined to the immediate area of the injection. In addition, one must also account for the necrotic needle tract that will accompany intraparenchymal injections. We have applied an experimental approach that locates the injection site approx 1 mm lateral to the inner boundary zone of the infarction and differentiates infarcted tissue by whole brain TTC staining (Linnik et al., 1995a). These injection coordinates allow for vector-driven protein expression in tissue that would normally die in the absence of intervention. The amount of viable tissue was determined by measuring the distance from the longitudinal fissure to the medial edge of the infarction at the injection site. Thus, one would predict that a protective therapy increases the amount of viable tissue at the injection site. Multiple measurements should be made with an accurate micrometer, rather than a ruler, to prevent distortion of the data related to the curvature of the brain.

5.1.4. Intraparenchymal Injection and Global Ischemia

This approach assumes that one is injecting the vector into the hippocampus near the CA1 region and attempting to determine an effect on neuronal survival after global ischemia. This experimental design poses significant technical challenges with the currently available vectors. However, Ho et al. (1995) have reported a bicistronic vector that efficiently expresses both the gene of interest and β-galactosidase as a reporter gene. Conceptually, this expression system allows one to directly identify neurons that are infected with the vectors (via β-galactosidase staining) and establish the effect of the gene of interest on the fate of the identified cell. This system permits quantitation by cell counting and has been shown to confer protection on cultured neurons in vitro (Ho et al., 1995). This clever approach has shown that overexpression of bcl-2 reduces cell death in global ischemia.

5.2. Transgenic Approaches to Gene Additions or Deletions

The ability to delete or amplify genes by transgenic methods offers a powerful approach for evaluating the function of apoptosis-related gene products in stroke. Two examples where this technology has contributed to understanding apoptosis in stroke include the antiapoptotic gene bcl-2 and the proapoptotic tumor suppressor gene p53. In the first example, Martinou et al. (1994) developed a transgenic animal that overexpressed bcl-2 and showed that these animals were relatively resistant to the effect of permanent ischemia induced by middle cerebral artery occlusion when compared to their wild-type controls.

The bcl-2 transgenic study showed that enhancing the function of an antiapoptotic gene can be protective in stroke. Similarly, deletion of a proapoptotic gene can also be protective. Crumrine et al. (1994) evaluated the effect of a p53 null mutation and observed that the null mutants developed smaller infarct than their wild-type controls. Interestingly, the heterozygous mutants produced smaller infarctions than the homozygous mutants, and both were smaller than the wild-type controls. Both studies support a role for apoptosis in ischemia-induced death and offer clues for understanding the pathophysiology and possible sites for pharmacologic intervention.

Although these initial studies are very promising, it has also become clear that the gene targets need to be considered carefully, particularly when they are a member of a larger gene family. For example, it was recently discovered that the mammalian homolog of ced-3 (a critical proapoptotic gene in *C. elegans*) was interleukin-1β converting enzyme (ICE), (Miura et al., 1993; Yuan et al., 1993). This led to the rapid development of transgenic ICE knockout animals (Kuida et al., 1995; Li et al., 1995e). Surprisingly, these animals exhibited very few overt developmental abnormalities. In addition, they exhibited normal apoptosis in most systems, with the notable exception being a defect in fas-mediated apoptosis.

One potential reason for this lack of an effect from ICE deletion in the transgenic mice became apparent when several mammalian homologs of the ICE gene were identified (Kumar, 1995). The discovery of these analogs suggested that ICE may have evolved several other members that play significant roles in mammalian apoptosis (Fernandes-Alnemri et al., 1994, 1995; Lazebnik et al., 1994; Wang et al., 1994; Nicholson et al., 1995; Tewari et al., 1995).

The lesson for those interested in applying transgenic technology to the study of neuronal apoptosis is that higher organisms often develop redundant mechanisms to accomplish the same fundamental tasks as the lower organisms. In practice, the first mammalian homolog of a cell death gene identified in simpler organisms like *C. elegans* often represents a single member of a family of genes in higher organisms.

A major consideration is that the addition or deletion of a gene in a transgenic animal can have unintended effects remote from its presumed function. Therefore, several experimental variables must be controlled before one can assign a cause and effect relationship between the genetic manipulation and the outcome variable. The remainder of this section will address the factors that should be considered when attempting to compare responses in transgenic animals to their nontransgenic littermates. The methodology necessary to develop transgenic animals will be considered beyond the scope of this review.

The process of generating transgenic animals can cause unintended consequences due to aberrations in development. The most obvious case occurs when the transgenic manipulation leads to nonviable offspring. However, when one is attempting to evaluate the effect of a genetic manipulation on infarct volume, one needs to determine that the cerebral circulation and autonomic response mechanisms have not been modified by the specific manipulation.

Several groups investigating transgenic animals in stroke models have identified parameters that should be evaluated prior to initiating a stroke study (Yang et al., 1994; Huang et al., 1994; Huang et al., 1995). First, one should determine that the gross brain cytoarchitecture has not been modified by the genetic manipulation. Typical observations might be to determine that brain volume, cortical volume, and subcortical structures all appear normal and equivalent to nontransgenic control animals.

Second, one should evaluate the cerebrovascular anatomy to ascertain that there are no gross differences in the circle of Willis or the major branching arteries. This can be accomplished by perfusing the animal with a 1% suspension of carbon black in India ink, and again compare transgenic animals to nontransgenic control animals (Ward et al., 1990).

Third, one should establish that the cardiovascular function is equivalent between transgenic and nontransgenic control animals. Obviously, changes in heart rate or blood pressure can change cerebral perfusion and impact the outcome after a stroke.

Fourth, one should consider establishing that the cerebral autoregulatory responses are not modified by the genetic manipulation. This can be evaluated by withdrawing arterial blood and measuring cerebral blood flow autoregulation by laser doppler flowmetry (Yang et al., 1994). The doppler flow determination involves the implantation of laser doppler probes for determination of regional cerebral blood flow. This approach should allow one to demonstrate that similar reductions in blood flow are measured in transgenic and nontransgenic controls and implies that the microvascular collateral circulation has not been altered.

Finally, one should generate data demonstrating that the genetic manipulation caused the intended change in function. These observations will be unique to the specific gene under investigation and will provide confidence that the gain of function or loss of function manipulation had the desired effect.

5.3. Future Directions

Many of the future directions for apoptosis research in cerebral ischemia are likely to be based on the application of discoveries from more readily manipulated systems, such as cell culture models and genetic models like *C. elegans* and *D. melanogaster*. For example, the analysis of the function, expression, and regulation of the extended gene families for the ced-3/ICE family of cysteine proteases (Martin and Green, 1995) and the ced-9/bcl-2 family of proteins (Nunez and Clarke, 1994) is proceeding in earnest in several laboratories. It will be particularly important to determine the specific substrates and functions of these gene products, as these areas are poorly understood. The initiating factors for apoptosis remain elusive, and signal transduction cascades that are employed in ischemia-induced apoptosis remain almost completely undefined. Intriguing information on the role of specific kinases and transcription factors in apoptotic PC-12 cells (Xia et al., 1995) suggest that the apoptosis cascade might be subject to factors that can potentiate or inhibit the process. Finally, there is good reason to be optimistic that these types of investigations will lead to novel, efficacious therapies for a devastating disease.

Acknowledgments

I would like to thank the many scientists that have contributed to our investigations regarding the role of apoptosis in ischemic neuronal death. In particular, I am deeply indebted to the following friends and colleagues: R. H. Zobrist, H. Federoff, J. Miller, S. Mehdi, P. Mason, M. Racke, F. Thompson, K. Schroeder and J. Koehl.

References

Akli S., Caillaud C., Vigne E., Stratford-Perricaudet L. D., Poenaru L., Perricaudet M., Kahn A., and Peschanski M. R. (1993) Transfer of a foreign gene into the brain using adenovirus vectors. *Nat. Genet.* **3,** 224–228.

Alles A., Alley K., Barrett J. C., Buttyan R., et al. (1991) Apoptosis: a general comment. *FASEB J.* **5,** 2127,2128.

Bajocchi G., Feldman S. H., Crystal R. G., and Mastrangeli A. (1993) Direct in vivo gene transfer to ependymal cells in the central nervous system using recombinant adenovirus vectors. *Nat. Genet.* **3,** 229–234.

Betz A. L., Yang G. Y., and Davidson B. L. (1995) Attenuation of stroke size in rats using an adenoviral vector to induce overexpression of interleukin-1 receptor antagonist in brain. *J. Cereb. Blood Flow Metab.* **15,** 547–551.

Buchan A. M. and Pulsinelli W. A. (1990) Hypothermia but not the N-methyl-D-aspartate antagonist, MK-801, attenuates neuronal damage in gerbils subjected to transient global ischemia. *Neuroscience* **10,** 311–316.

Charriaut-Marlangue C., Margaill I., Plotkine M., and Ben-Ari Y. (1995) Early endonuclease activation following reversible focal ischemia in the rat brain. *J. Cereb. Blood Flow Metab.* **15,** 385–388.

Chen S. T., Hsu C. Y., Hogan E. L., Maricq H., and Balentine J. D. (1986) A model of focal ischemic stroke in the rat: reproducible extensive cortical infarction. *Stroke* **4,** 738–743.

Crumrine R. C., Thomas A. L., and Morgan P. F. (1994) Attenuation of p53 expression protects against focal ischemic damage in transgenic mice. *J. Cereb. Blood Flow Metab.* **14,** 887–891.

Darzynkiewicz Z., Bruno S., Del Bino G., Gorczyca W., Hotz M. A., Lassota P., and Traganos F. (1992) Features of apoptotic cells measured by flow cytometry *Cytometry* **13,** 795–808.

Deckworth T. L. and Johnson E. M. (1993) Temporal events associated with programmed cell death (apoptosis) of sympathetic neurons deprived of nerve growth factor. *J. Cell Biol.* **123,** 1207–1222.

Deshpande J., Bergstedt K., Linden T., Kalimo H., and Wieloch T. (1992) Ultrastructural changes in the hippocampal CA1 region following transient cerebral ischemia: evidence against programmed cell death. *Exp. Brain Res.* **88,** 91–105.

Dive C., Gregory C. D., Phipps D. J., Evans D. L., Milner A. E., and Wyllie A. H. (1992) Analysis and discrimination of necrosis and apoptosis (programmed cell death) by multiparameter flow cytometry. *Biochem. Biophys. Acta* **1133,** 275–285.

Fernandes-Alnemri T. Litwack G., and Alnemri E. S. (1994) CPP32, a novel human apoptotic protein with homology to *Caenorhabditis elegans* cell death protein Ced-3 and mammalian interleukin-1 beta-converting enzyme. *J. Biol. Chem.* **269,** 30,761–30,764.

Fernandes-Alnemri T., Litwack G., and Alnemri E. S. (1993) Mch2, a new member of the apoptotic Ced-3/Ice cysteine protease gene family. *Cancer Res.* **55,** 2737–2742.

Gavrieli Y., Sherman Y., and Ben-Sasson S. A. (1992) Identification of programmed cell death *in situ* via specific labeling of nuclear DNA fragmentation. *J. Cell Biol.* **119,** 493–501.

Gibellini D., Zauli G., Re C. M., Furlini G., Lolli S., Bassini A., Celeghini C., and La Placa M. (1995) *In situ* polymerase chain reaction technique revealed by flow cytometry as a tool for gene detection. *Anal. Biochem.* **228,** 252–258.

Ginsberg M. D., Sternau L. L., Globus M. Y.-T., Dietrich W. D., and Busto R. (1992) Therapeutic modulation of brain temperature: relevance to ischemic brain injury. *Cerebrovascular and Brain Metab. Rev.* **4,** 189–225.

Heron A., Pollard H., Dessi F., Moreau J., Lasbennes F., Ben-Ari Y., and Charriaut-Marlangue C. (1993) Regional variability in DNA fragmentation after global ischemia evidenced by combined histological and gel electrophoresis observations in the rat brain. *J. Neurochem.* **61,** 1973–1976.

Ho D. Y., Saydam T. C., Fink S. L., Lawrence M. S., and Sapolsky R. M. (1995) Defective herpes simplex virus vectors expressing the rat brain glucose transporter protect cultured neurons from necrotic insults. *J. Neurochem.* **65,** 842–850.

Hossmann K.-A. (1993) Viability thresholds and the penumbra of focal ischemia. *Ann. Neurol.* **36,** 557–565.

Hsu C. Y., He Y. Y., Lin T. N., Wu G., and Marangos P. J. (1992) Stroke models for preclinical trials of neuroprotective agents, in *Emerging Strategies in Neuroprotection,* Marangos, H., ed., Birkhaeuser, Boston, MA, pp. 44–56.

Huang Z., Huang P. L., Panahian N., Dalkara T., Fishman M. C., and Moskowitz M. A. (1994) Effects of cerebral ischemia in mice deficient in neuronal nitric oxide synthase. *Science* **265,** 1883–1885.

Huang P. L. Huang Z., Mashimo H., Bloch K. D., Moskowitz M. A., Bevan J. A., and Fishman M. C. (1995) Hypertension in mice lacking the gene for endothelial nitric oxide synthase. *Nature* **377,** 239–242.

Hunter A. J., Green A. R., and Cross A. J. (1995) Animals models of acute ischaemic stroke: can they predict clinically successful neuroprotective drugs? *Trends Pharmacol. Sci.* **16,** 123–128.

Islam N., Aftabuddin M., Moriwaki A., and Hori Y. (1995) Detection of DNA damage induced by apoptosis in the rat brain following incomplete ischemia. *Neurosci. Lett.* **188,** 159–162.

Kerr J. F. R., Wyllie A. H., and Currie A. R. (1972) Apoptosis: a basic biological phenomenon with wide ranging implications in tissue kinetics. *Br. J. Cancer* **26,** 239–257.

Kerr J. F., Gobe G. C., Winterford C. M., and Harmon B. V. (1995) Anatomical methods in cell death. *Methods Cell Biol.* **46,** 1–27.

Kirino T. (1982) Delayed neuronal death in the gerbil hippocampus following ischemia *Brain Res.* **239,** 57–69.

Kothari R. U., Brott T., Broderick J. P., and Hamilton C. A. (1995) Emergency physicians: accuracy in the diagnosis of stroke. *Stroke* **26,** 2238–2241.

Krajewski S., Mai J. K., Sikorska M., Mossakowski M. J., and Reed J. C. (1995) Upregulation of Bax protein levels in neurons following cerebral ischemia. *J. Neurosci.* **15,** 6364–6376.

Kuida K., Lippke J. A., Ku G., Harding M. W., Livingston D. J., Su M. S.-S., and Flavell R. A. (1995) Altered cytokine export and apoptosis in mice deficient in interleukin-1β converting enzyme. *Science* **267,** 2000–2003.

Kumar S. (1995) ICE-like proteases in apoptosis. *Trends Biochem. Sci.* **20,** 198–202.

Lazebnik Y. A., Kaufmann S. H., Desnoyers S., Poirier G. G., and Earnshaw W. C. (1994) Cleavage of poly(ADP-ribose) polymerase by a proteinase with properties like ICE. *Nature* **371,** 346,347.

Li Y., Chopp M., Zhang Z. G., Zaloga C., Niewenhuis L., and Gautam S. (1994) p53-Immunoreactive protein and p53 mRNA expression after transient middle cerebral artery occlusion in rats. *Stoke* **25,** 849–856.

Li Y., Chopp M., Jiang N., Yao F., and Zaloga C. (1995a) Temporal profile of *in situ* DNA fragmentation after transient middle cerebral artery occlusion in the rat. *J. Cereb. Blood Flow Metab.* **15,** 389–397.

Li Y., Chopp M., Jiang N., Zhang Z. G., and Zaloga C. (1995b) Induction of DNA fragmentation after 10 to 120 minutes of focal cerebral ischemia in rats. *Stroke* **26,** 1252–1258.

Li Y., Sharov V. G., Jiang N., Zaloga C., Sabbah H. N., and Chopp M. (1995c) Ultrastructural and light microscopic evidence of apoptosis after middle cerebral artery occlusion in the rat. *Am. J. Pathol.* **146,** 1045–1051.

Li Y., Chopp M., Jiang N., and Zaloga C. (1995d) *In situ* detection of DNA fragmentation after focal cerebral ischemia in mice. *Mol. Brain Res.* **28,** 164–168.

Li P., Allen H., Banerjee S., Franklin S., Herzog L., Johnston C., McDowell J., Paskind M., Rodman L., Salfeld J., Towne E., Tracey D., Wardwell S., Wei F., Wong W., Kamen R., and Seshadri T. (1995e) Mice deficient in IL-1 beta-converting enzyme are defective in production of mature IL-1 beta and resistant to endotoxic shock. *Cell* **80,** 401–411.

Linnik M. D., Hatfield M. D., Swope M. D., and Ahmed N. K. (1993a) Induction of programmed cell death in a dorsal root ganglia x neuroblastoma cell line. *J. Neurobiol.* **24,** 433–446.

Linnik M. D., Zobrist R. H., and Hatfield M. D. (1993b) Evidence supporting a role for programmed cell death in focal cerebral ischemia in rats. *Stroke* **24,** 2002–2009.

Linnik M. D., Zahos P., Geschwind M. D., and Federoff H. J. (1995a) Expression of bcl-2 from a defective herpes simplex virus 1 vector limits neuronal death in focal cerebral ischemia. *Stroke* **26,** 1670–1675.

Linnik M. D., Miller J. A., Sprinkle-Cavallo J., Mason P. J., Thompson F. Y., Montgomery L. R., and Schroeder K. K. (1995b) Apoptotic DNA fragmentation in the rat cerebral cortex induced by permanent middle cerebral artery occlusion. *Mol. Brain Res.* **32**, 116–124.

MacManus J. P., Buchan A. M., Hill I. E., Rasquinha I., and Preston E. (1993) Global ischemia can cause DNA fragmentation indicative of apoptosis in rat brain. *Neurosci. Lett.* **164**, 89–92.

MacManus J. P., Hill I. E., Huang Z.-G., Rasquinha I., Xue D., and Buchan A. M. (1994) DNA damage consistent with apoptosis in transient focal ischemic neocortex *Neuroreport* **5**, 493–496.

MacManus J. P., Hill I. E., Preston E., Rasquinha I., Walker T., and Buchan A. M. (1995) Differences in DNA fragmentation following transient cerebral or decapitation ischemia in rats. *J. Cereb. Blood Flow Metab.* **15**, 728–737.

Manev H., Kharlamov A., and Armstrong D. M. (1994) Photochemical brain injury in rats triggers DNA fragmentation, p53 and HSP72. *NeuroReport* **5**, 2661–2664.

Martin D. P., Schmidt R. E., DiStefano P. S., Lowry O. H., Carter J. G., and Johnson E. M. (1988) Inhibitors of protein synthesis and RNA synthesis prevent neuronal death caused by nerve growth factor deprivation. *J. Cell Biol.* **106**, 829–844.

Martin D. P., Ito A., Horigome K., Lampe P. A., and Johnson E. M. (1993) Biochemical characterization of programmed cell death in NGF-deprived sympathetic neurons. *J. Neurobiol.* **23**, 1205–1220.

Martin S. J. and Green D. R. (1995) Protease activation during apoptosis: death by a thousand cuts? *Cell* **82**, 349–352.

Martinou J. C., Dubois-Dauphin M., Staple J. K., Rodriguez I., Frankowski H., Missotten M., Albertini P., Talabot D., Catsicas S., Pietra C., and Huarte J. (1994) Overexpression of BCL-2 in transgenic mice protects neurons from naturally occurring cell death and experimental ischemia. *Neuron* **13**, 1017–1030.

Miura M., Zhu H., Rotello R., Hartwieg E. A., and Yuan J. (1993) Induciton of apoptosis in fibroblasts by IL-1β-converting enzyme, a mammalian homolog of the *C. elegans* cell death gene ced-3. *Cell* **75**, 653–660.

Mossakowski M. J., Hiligier W., and Januszewski S. (1986) Morphological abnormalities in the CNS of rats in experimental postresuscitation period. *Neuropathol. Pol.* **24**, 471–489.

Nitatori T., Sato N., Waguri S., Karasawa Y., Araki H., Shibanai K., Kominami E., and Uchiyama Y. (1995) Delayed neuronal death in the CA1 pyramidal cell layer of the gerbil hippocampus following transient ischemia is apoptosis. *J. Neurosci.* **15**, 1001–1011.

Nicholson D. W., Ali A., Thornberry N. A., Vaillancourt J. P., Ding C. K., Gallant M., Gareau Y., Griffin P. R., Labelle M., Lazebnik Y. A., Munday N. A., Raju S. M., Smulson M. E., Yamin T.-T., Yu V. L., and Miller D. K. (1995) Identification and inhibition of the ICE/Ced-3 protease necessary for mammalian apoptosis *Nature* **376,** 37–43.

Nunez G. and Clarke M. F. (1994) The bcl-2 family of proteins: regulators of cell death and survival. *Trends Cell Biol.* **4,** 399–403.

Okamoto M., Matsumoto M., Ohtsuki T., Taguchi A., Mikoshiba K., Yanagihara T., and Kamada T. (1993) Internucleosomal DNA cleavage involved in ischemia-induced neuronal death. *Biochem. Biophys. Res. Comm.* **196,** 1356–1362.

Oppenheim R. W. (1991) Cell death during development of the nervous system. *Ann. Rev. Neurosci.* **14,** 453–501.

Pandey S., Walker P. R., and Sikorska M. (1994) Separate pools of endonuclease activity are responsible for internucleosomal and high molecular mass DNA fragmentation during apoptosis. *Biochem. Cell Biol.* **72,** 625–629.

Papas S., Crepel V., Hasboun D., Jorquera I., Chinestra P., and Ben-Ari Y. (1992) Cycloheximide reduces the effects of anoxic insult in vivo and in vitro. *Eur. J. Neurosci.* **4,** 758–765.

Park C. K., Mendelow A. D., Graham D. I., McCulloch J., and Teasdale G. M. (1988) Correlation of triphenyltetrazolium chloride perfusion staining with conventional neurohistology in the detection of early brain ischemia. *Neuropathol. Appl. Neurobiol.* **14,** 289–298.

Pechan P. A., Yoshida T., Panahian N., Moskowitz M. A., and Breakfield X. O. (1995) Genetically modified fibroblasts producing NGF protect hippocampal neurons after ischemia in the rat. *NeuroReport* **6,** 669–672.

Pulsinelli W. A. and Brierley J. B. (1979) A new model of bilateral hemispheric ischemia in the unanesthetized rat. *Stroke* **10,** 267–272.

Pulsinelli W. A., Brierley J. B., and Plum F. (1982) Temporal profile of neuronal damage in a model of transient forebrain ischemia. *Ann. Neurol.* **11,** 491–499.

Pulsinelli W. (1992) Pathophysiology of acute ischemic stroke. *Lancet* **339,** 533–536.

Sacco R. L. (1994) Classification of stroke, in *Clinical Atlas of Cerebrovascular Disorders,* Fischer M., ed., Mosby-Year Book Europe, London, England, pp. 2.3–2.23.

Schwartz L. M., Smith S. W., Jones M. E. E., and Osborne B. A. (1993) Do all programmed cell deaths occur via apoptosis? *Proc. Natl. Acad. Sci. USA* **90,** 980–984.

Sei Y., Von Lubitz K. J., Basile A. S., Borner M. M., Lin R. C., Skolnick P., and Fossom L. H. (1994) Internucleosomal DNA fragmentation in gerbil hippocampus following forebrain ischemia. *Neurosci. Lett.* **171,** 179–182.

Shigeno T., Yamasaki Y., Kato G., Kausaka K., Mima T., Takakura K., Graham D. I., and Furukawa S. (1990) Reduction of delayed neuronal death by inhibition of protein synthesis. *Neurosci. Lett.* **120,** 117–119.

Shigeno T., Mima T., Takakura K., Graham D. I., Kato G., Hashimoto Y., and Furukawa S. (1991) Amelioration of delayed neuronal death in the hippocampus by nerve growth factor. *J. Neurosci.* **11,** 2914–2919.

Tewari M., Quan L. T., O'Rourke K., Desnoyers S., Zeng. Z., Beidler D. R., Poirier G. G., Salvesen G. S., and Dixit V. M. (1995) Yama/CPP32 beta, a mammalian homolog of CeD-3, is a CrmA-inhibitable protease that cleaves the death substrate poly(ADP-ribose) polymerase. *Cell* **81,** 801–809.

Tominaga T., Kure S., Narisawa K., and Yoshimoto T. (1993) Endonuclease activation following focal ischemic injury in the rat brain. *Brain Res.* **608,** 21–26.

Tulleken C. A. F. and Abraham J. (1975) The influence of changes in arterial CO_2 and blood pressure on the collateral circulation and the regional perfusion pressure in monkeys with occlusion of the middle cerebral artery. *Acta Neurochirurgica* **32,** 161–173.

Walker P. R., Kokileva L., LeBlanc J., and Sikorska M. (1993) Detection of the initial stages of DNA fragmentation in apoptosis. *Biotechniques* **5,** 1032–1040.

Walker P. R., Weaver V. M., Lach B., LeBlanc J., and Sikorska M. (1994) Endonuclease activities associated with high molecular weight and internucleosomal DNA fragmentation in apoptosis. *Exp. Cell Res.* **213,** 100–106.

Wang L., Miura M., Bergeron L., Zhu H., and Yuan J. (1994) Ich-1, an Ice/ced-3-related gene, encodes both positive and negative regulators of programmed cell death. *Cell* **78,** 739–750.

Ward R., Collins R. L., Tanguay G., and Miceli D. (1990) A quantitative study of cerebrovascular variation in inbred mice. *J. Anat.* **173,** 87–95.

Watson D. B., Dietrich W. D., Busto R., Wachte M. S., and Ginsburg M. D. (1985) Induction of reproducible brain infarction by photochemically initiated thrombosis. *Ann. Neurol.* **17,** 497–504.

Wyllie A. H., Kerr J. F. R., and Currie A. R. (1980) Cell death, the significance of apoptosis. *Int. Rev. Cytol.* **68,** 251–306.

Xia Z., Dickens M., Raingeaud J., Davis R. J., and Greenberg M. E. (1995) Opposing effects of ERK and JNK-p38 MAP kinases on apoptosis. *Science* **270,** 1326–1331.

Yamamoto S., Yoshimine T., Fujita T., Kuroda R., Irie T., Fujioka K., and Hayakawa T. (1992) Protective effect of NGF atelocollagen minipellet on the hippocampal delayed neuronal death in gerbils. *Neurosci. Lett.* **141,** 161–165.

Yang G., Chan P. H., Chen J., Carlson E., Chen S. F., Weinstein P., Epstein C. J., and Kamii H. (1994) Human copper-zinc superoxide dismutase transgenic mice are highly resistant to reperfusion injury after focal cerebral ischemia *Stroke* **25,** 165–170.

Yip P. K., He Y. Y., Hsu C. Y., Garg N., Marangos P., and Hogan E. L. (1991) Effect of plasma glucose on infarct size in focal cerebral ischemia-reperfusion *Neurology* **41,** 899–905.

Yuan Y., Shaham S., Ledoux S., Ellis H. M., and Horvitz H. R. (1993) The *C. elegans* cell death gene ced-3 encodes a protein similar to mammalian interleukin-1β-converting enzyme. *Cell* **75,** 641–652.

Analyses of Apoptosis-Associated DNA Fragmentation In Vivo During Neurodegeneration of the Peripheral Olfactory System in Adult Mammals

Emmanuel Moyse and Denis Michel

1. Introduction

1.1. Apoptotic DNA Fragmentation

DNA fragments of discrete sizes, multiples of monomeric units, have clearly been observed during the period of nuclear degeneration of the terminal lens cell differentiation (Appleby and Modak, 1977). The same puzzling phenomenon has been associated with thymocyte apoptoses (Wyllie, 1980) and rapidly generalized to a wide variety of experimental or natural cases of programmed cell death. By contrast with necrosis, which is a passive lysis of cells following disruption of membrane integrity under external aggressions, programmed cell death involves the specific triggering of stereotyped active processes with *de novo* gene expression (Ellis et al., 1991; Schwartz, 1991). Ultrastructure of most mammalian cells undergoing programmed cell death was observed to change similary through membrane blebbing, chromatin condensation, and genesis of apoptotic bodies (Kerr et al., 1972), along with internucleosomal DNA fragmentation (Wyllie, 1980). This common sequence of events led to a concept of apopto-

From: *Neuromethods, Vol. 29: Apoptosis Techniques and Protocols*
Ed: J. Poirier Humana Press Inc.

sis and to the supposition that all programmed cell deaths could occur via apoptosis (Wyllie, 1980). Currently, many authors use the terms "programmed cell death" and "apoptosis" interchangeably. However, such assimilation has been recently challenged by the biochemical and ultrastructural investigation of one among the longest recognized models of programmed cell death: the ecdysone-dependent autolysis of intersegmental muscles during metamorphosis in moths (Lockshin and William, 1965). The pattern of cell death displayed by this insect pupal organ was found to differ from apoptotic T-cells of mammals by cell-surface morphology, nuclear ultrastructure, gene expression, and absence of DNA internucleosomal fragmentation (Schwartz et al., 1993). It appears, therefore, that some eukaryotic cells may use a programmed cell death mechanism that is distinct from apoptosis (Schwartz et al., 1993). Necrosis should then be opposed to programmed cell death, one mechanism of which, among others, is apoptosis.

Nonetheless, the cleavage of genomic DNA into nucleosome-sized fragments, multiples of 180–200 bp, is now considered a specific hallmark of apoptosis. Molecular mechanisms underlying this irreversible cellular activity are not elucidated, but are assumed to involve a Ca^{2+}- and Mg^{2+}-dependent endonuclease activity that could be ensured by DNase I (Peitsch et al., 1993b). The apoptotic DNA fragmentation is not due to double-strand cuts, but is the result of frequent single-strand breaks (Peitsch et al., 1993a; Tomei et al., 1993). As a consequence, before appearance of DNA fragments in cells undergoing apoptosis, a growing number of nicks accumulate in DNA, still appearing of high molecular weight in nondenaturing electrophoresis gels. Hence, labeling DNA nicks is likely to reveal earliest stages of apoptotic DNA degradation, but also to increase the noise by labeling DNA breaks unrelated to apoptosis.

The precise involvement of DNA fragmentation in apoptosis is still controversial. Whether it is causally related to cell death (Brüne et al., 1991), or is a dispensable consequence of cell death (Ucker et al., 1992; Schwartz et al., 1993) remains an open question. Nevertheless, because of its technical simplicity, the detection of DNA fragmentation is now widely used as a rapid way to assess the presence of apoptoses and to quantify them with more accuracy than morphological criteria, which may be difficult and confusing in routine histological sections (Wijsman et al., 1993). In addition, the criterion of DNA ladderization is restricted to apoptotic cell deaths, contrary to the cytotoxicity assays like the release of cytoplasmic enzymes. Here, we focus our attention on two main methods of in vivo detection of DNA fragmentation, using as a neuronal model of apoptosis the peripheral olfactory system of adult mouse. These methods are: observation of "ladders" after electrophoresis of genomic DNA; and *in situ* detection of apoptotic nuclei by labeling DNA ends. The latter method permits precise localization of apoptotic cell populations at the light microscopic level. The former permits unambiguous establishment of the apoptotic nature of DNA breaks, by comparison, for example, with necrotic DNA degradations. Electrophoretic bands corresponding to internucleosomal DNA fragments of various sizes can be visualized by mere ethidium bromide staining of gels. However, visualization of apoptotic DNA fragmentation is greatly facilitated by radioactive or colorimetric labeling of DNA breaks prior to electrophoresis (Rösl, 1992). DNA end-labeling on paraffin sections of fixed organs has also allowed *in situ* detection of apoptotic cell nuclei (Gavrieli et al., 1992) more specifically than by conventional histology at the light microscopic level (Kerr et al., 1987; Wijsman et al., 1993). *In situ* labeling of DNA ends has greatly increased the probability of detecting apoptoses. Apoptotic cell appearance is indeed limited to only a few minutes, whereas the period through which dying cells can be revealed by labeling DNA breaks has been kinetically estimated to be between 1 and 3 h. Apoptotic bodies could reportedly be detected a few hours before they are phagocytized (Brush et al., 1990; Wyllie et al., 1980), but technical constraints make electron microscopic assessment of tissue ultrastructure much more restricted spatially than light microscopy.

1.2. Neuronal DNA Fragmentation

Assessments of genomic DNA fragmentations have allowed researchers to conclude that neuronal degeneration can also proceed through apoptotic mechanisms. Neuronal apoptosis programs are clearly triggered in cultured neurones after growth factor withdrawal (Estus et al., 1994; Greenlund et al., 1995) or after addition of amyloid protein fragments (Forloni et al., 1993; Loo et al., 1993), as well as in vivo, by excitotoxic amino acids (Kure et al., 1991; Filipkowski et al., 1994) or ischemia (MacManus et al., 1993). The examination of spontaneous DNA fragmentation *in situ* during development has revealed that neuronal deaths occur prior to synaptogenesis, perhaps in relation to the regulation of the neuron cell number (Wood et al., 1993). We observed that the retrograde neurodegeneration of olfactory sensory neurons, consequent to ablation of their synaptic target, is the result of a near synchronized induction of apoptotic programs (Michel et al., 1994). In this case, the visualization of apoptosis-associated DNA fragmentation in neurones has brought about a concrete substrate to the old concept of target-induced neuronal survival.

2. DNA End-Labeling Procedures

The labeling of DNA ends strongly increases the sensitivity of detection of apoptotic DNA fragmentation by electrophoresis (Tilly and Hsueh, 1993), thus reducing the amounts of tissues required for this analysis. It is also valuable for discriminating *in situ* the apoptotic nuclei, containing numerous DNA ends, from intact ones. The internucleosomal single-strand cuts are assumed to occur randomly; hence, the resulting double-strand breaks are expected to belong to all three possible categories: blunt, 5'-protruding, and 3'-protruding ends. Since the cellular enzymatic activity responsible for the apoptotic DNA fragmentation yields 5'-phosphate and 3'-OH ends, experimental procedures most often selected in the literature use the extension of 3' termini by DNA polymerases. Several enzymes are potentially good candidates for this purpose (Table 1). Although they can label these different DNA ends with various efficiencies, most of them are convenient because labeling only a subpopulation of DNA breaks is sufficient to reveal DNA fragmentation.

DNA-dependent DNA polymerases are expected to display different 3' end labeling activities, depending on the presence of all four nucleotide precursors (Table 1). In most cases for example, the Klenow fragment of the *E. coli*, DNA polymerase I cannot label the blunt or 3'-protruding ends in the presence of a radiolabeled nuleotide if the three others are present. This problem can be circumvented by adding only the radiolabeled nucleotide in the incubation buffer. In this way, the processing activity of the enzyme will allow it to reach the first nucleotide corresponding to the radiolabeled one, in each 3' end of DNA fragments. In the presence of all nucleotide precursors, the *E. coli* DNA polymerase I displays a high nick translation activity. However, by allowing very efficient incorporations of radiolabeled nucleotides at every DNA nick, this method is likely to increase the background of DNA labeling. For the same reason, the template-independent DNA polymerase terminal deoxynucleotidyl transferase (TdT) deserves special attention since it can label doublestrand, but not single-strand breaks. This feature turns out to be useful in the present case, by avoiding the labeling of DNA nicks sometimes unrelated to apoptosis. The labeling of 5' protruding ends by TdT is possible in particular experimental conditions, but is not necessary in the present case. Besides, TdT can add several labeled nucleotides at 3' ends of DNA, further increasing the efficiency of labeling *in situ*. For ladder detections, however, the TdT-polymerized tails can modify the sizes of oligonucleosomal fragments; so it may be useful to preclude such polymerizations by adding chain-terminating dideoxynucleotides (Tilly and Hsueh, 1993).

3. The DNA Ladderization

Contrary to the mere presence of DNA ends inside nuclei, the presence of oligonucleosomal DNA fragmentation is an

Table 1
DNA Break Labeling Activities of Template-Dependent (A. B. C, D, E)
and Template-Independent (F) DNA Polymerases

		A DNA pol 1	B Klenow	C T4 pol T7 pol	D R.T. Mod. T7 pol	E exo⁻ therm. pol	F TdT
5' → 3' exonuclease activity		+	−	+	−	+	−
3' → 5' exonuclease activity		+	+	++	−	−	−
Displacement of strand ↓		+	+	−	−	−	−
═ ═ : ───────── : nick ═ ═ : ─── : ─────		+ (+)	+ (+/−)	+ (−)	− (−)	− (+)	− (−)
DNA break	5' protruding ═ ═ : ─── : ───── ═ ═ : ───	+ (+/−)	+ (+/−)	+ (+/−)	− (+/−)	− (+/−)	− (−)
	3' protruding ═ ═ : ─── : ───── ═ ═ : ───	+ (−)	+ (−)	+ (−)	− (−)	− (−)	+ (+)
	blunt ═ ═ : ─── : ───── ═ ═ : ───	+ (−)	+ (−)	+ (−)	− (−)	− (−)	+ (+)

The indicated labeling activities are obtained in presence of a single-labeled nucleotide, either alone (without parentheses), or in presence of the three other cold ones (in parentheses). The labeling activities of 5' protruding termini by the two first categories of enzymes, DNA pol I, and Klenow fragment, in the presence of the four nucleotide precursors including a single-labeled one, depends on the presence or absence of nucleotides complementary to this labeled one in the single-stranded ends, and then is more probable with long 5' protruding termini. In the presence of a single-labeled nucleotide out of four, the A, B, and C categories can only label an average of one-fourth of blunt and 3' protruding ends, and for this reason, have been indicated (−). The same feature is observed for D and E categories, in the presence of a single-labeled nucleotide. It is also noteworthy that TdT can, to some extent, be rendered able to label 5' protruding ends if Co²⁺ is added as a cofactor. DNA pol I: E. coli DNA polymerase I. Klenow: large, or Klenow, fragment of the E. coli DNA polymerase I. R.T.: reverse transcriptase. Mod. T7 pol: modified T7 DNA polymerase (Sequenase™ and Sequenase version 2.0). Exo⁻ therm. DNA pol: 3' → 5' exonuclease⁻ thermostable DNA polymerase (like Taq DNA polymerase). TdT: terminal deoxynucleotidyl transferase.

unambiguous proof of apoptosis. But in turn, absence of DNA ladders does not rule out occurrence of apoptotic cells, since the generalization of DNA fragmentation in all apoptotic processes remains to be definitively established. Monitoring DNA ladders, when detectable, can serve both to identify and to quantify apoptoses. The visualization of DNA ladders is simple in its principle, based on the electrophoretic separation of genomic DNA fragments extracted from cultured cells or crude tissues. If only a small fraction of the cellular population undergoes apoptosis, the end labeling of DNA fragments markedly improves their detection (Rosl, 1992). Finally, quantifying DNA ladders permits comparison of the apoptosis intensity between different biological conditions or tissue samples.

3.1. Nucleic Acids Extraction

3.1.1. Rapid Extraction of DNA from Tissues

Standard methods of DNA preparation (Ausubel et al., 1994) are convenient. In addition, preparations can be enriched in DNA fragments by omitting the treatment of chromatin by proteinase K (Peitsch et al., 1993a) or by using extraction methods for low molecular weight DNA (Hirt, 1967). It is worth noting that, because of the early breakdown of nuclear membrane in apoptotic cells, DNA fragments can either be present in cytoplasm or can be released from cells and thus detected in the incubating medium (Joseph et al., 1993). An RNA contamination should be eliminated because it can interfere with the following steps of the procedure. This elimination can be carried out by two ways: If the DNA precipitate is obtained by centrifugation, the pellet should then be treated with RNase A, reextracted and reprecipitated before dosage; if the DNA precipitate is visible after ethanol addition, it can easily be removed with a stick and transferred into a new tube, the RNA precipitates remaining in the former tube. Experience shows that, contrary to former expectations, small oligonucleosomal fragments coprecipitate with high molecular weight DNA. One must keep in mind, however, that a minimum of 10 mg of fresh tissue is necessary to obtain a visible precipitate.

3.1.2. Simultaneous Extraction of DNA and RNA

This may be useful in many cases, for monitoring the variations of some mRNA levels in relation to the onset of DNA fragmentation. This approach would permit, for instance, checking for the possible involvement of particular genes in the apoptotic genetic program, as already demonstrated in neuronal apoptoses for c-*fos* (Smeyne et al., 1993; Michel et al., 1994), c-*Jun* (Estus et al., 1994), or cyclin D1 (Freeman et al., 1994). Thanks to the high sensitivity of reverse transcription-mediated polymerase chain reactions, very small amounts of RNA are sufficient for such purposes. Ideally, the separated preparation of DNA and RNA can be achieved through the preliminary isolation of nuclei containing DNA from cytoplasm that bear mature mRNAs. Starting from cultured cells, such rough cellular fractionation can easily be carried out by gentle treatment with detergents like Nonidet P-40 (Sambrook et al., 1989). However, this method is no longer practicable when studying apoptoses in vivo, as in the present example in olfactory turbinates of adult mammals. In this case, all nucleic acids are extracted simultaneously from freshly dissected tissues; DNA and RNA are thereafter separated by differential precipitation (Michel et al., 1994).

3.2. Visualization of DNA Ladders

The mere incorporation of fluorescent DNA intercalators, such as ethidium, is fully sufficient for visualizing laddering patterns in most cases of massive and synchronous apoptoses. The best examples are provided by models of leukocyte apoptoses (Wyllie, 1980). However, in tissues or cell populations in which apoptotic cells are in the minority, the ethidium bromide staining should be replaced by a labeling of DNA ends. By increasing the sensitivity of detection, ladder labeling procedures permit starting from as little as 100 μg of tissue.

In addition, contrary to ethidium-UV fluorescence, the visualization of ladders after end labeling has the great advantage of yielding signals quantitatively related to the number of molecules, but not to their molecular weight. Con-

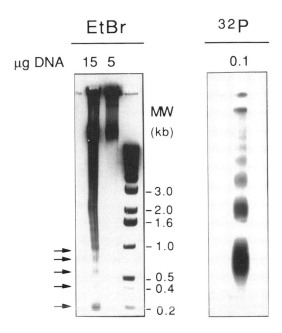

Fig. 1. Comparative visualizations of DNA ladders after ethidium staining and radioactive end-labeling. Aliquots of the same DNA from targetless olfactory turbinates have been electrophoresed through 1% (left panel) or 2% (right panel) agarose gels, either without (left panel) or after ^{32}P-end labeling (right panel). The untreated DNA is visualized by ethidium-UV staining and the ^{32}P-labeled DNA by radioautography. The radioactive labeling procedure both yields more distinct laddering patterns and requires a lower amount of DNA than the other one.

sequently, end labeling methods reveal short and long DNA fragments with equal intensity. Figure 1 presents the two different analyses of the same genomic DNA, extracted from mouse olfactory mucosa 32 h after bulbectomy. On the ethidium-stained gel, visualization of DNA ladders requires as much as 15 µg of genomic DNA, and even in these conditions only the smallest fragments can be visualized. The high molecular weight DNA, present in excess, saturates the gel and creates a smear that hinders the visibility of ladders. By contrast, a radioautogram of 100 ng of the same DNA, after radioactive end labeling and gel electrophoresis, displays a distinct laddering pattern (Fig. 1, right panel).

3.3. Electrophoretic Separation of DNA Fragments

Standard horizontal Tris-acetate or Tris-borate agarose gels (Sambrook et al., 1989) are fully adequate for separating oligonucleosomes of different sizes. A high agarose concentration (2–3%) and a relatively short distance of migration are favorable parameters for maintaining a thin appearance to the bands of oligonucleosomal fragments. Indeed, the rungs of DNA ladders are not bands of discrete sizes but are made up of populations of DNA fragments very heterogeneous in size (Peitsch et al., 1993a). This heterogeneity may have been further increased by the enzymatic labeling step.

A fraction of the labeling reactions can be loaded directly onto the gel, since the unincorporated nucleotides migrate rapidly in the front of electrophoresis. Care should be taken, in the case of radioactive labeling, to discard the fraction of the gel containing free nucleotides in the bin for radioactivity.

After vacuum drying, the gels are exposed onto X-ray films for time periods ranging from a few minutes to several hours, depending on the intensity of signals. Too lengthy time exposures can reveal a background of DNA laddering in the cellular population that does not account for the studied cellular responses.

3.4. Quantification of Apoptoses via DNA Ladder Analysis

If apoptotic cells are not too diluted relative to the healthy ones within the tissue extract, one may expect that the ratio DNA ladders/total DNA would give an estimation of cell death intensity in a given tissue. Quantitative analyses however, are relatively delicate since they rely upon the careful quantification of genomic DNA prior to the DNA end labeling. In addition, to ensure similar labeling efficiencies of all DNA samples, labeling reactions should be carried out simultaneously, using a premix containing radiolabeled nucleotides and enzyme (Table 2, B). Finally, aliquots of the labeling reactions containing identical amounts of DNA should be electrophoresed in parallel through the same gel.

Table 2
Rapid Procedure for Visualization and Quantification of DNA Ladders

DNA extraction from crude tissues

1. Scant crushing of the tissue under liquid nitrogen.
2. Lysis in lysis buffer (100 mM NaCl, 100 mM Tris-HCl, pH 8.0, 50 mM EDTA and 1% sodium dodecylsulfate.
3. Addition of 1 mg/mL proteinase K and incubation overnight at 55°C.
4. Extraction with phenol/chloroform and ethanol precipitation.
5. RNA degradation in presence of 10 µg/mL of boiled RNase A.
6. Extraction with phenol/chloroform and ethanol precipitation.
7. Dissolution and careful quantification of DNA by absorbance at 260 nm.

   Note: If the DNA precipitate is visible after ethanol addition at the step 4, it can be picked up with a rod without centrifugation and transferred into a novel tube without centrifugation. This method avoids a subsequent treatment with RNase A.

Labeling DNA ladders using the Klenow polymerase

1. Transfert 1 µg of each DNA to be tested in a new tube, complete with H_2O to 5 µL.
2. Add rapidly to each tube 15 µL of a premix as follows:

   Premix for 10 labeling reactions:

H_2O	126 µL
10X Medium salt buffer (Sambrook et al., 1989)	20 µL
[$\alpha-^{32}P$] dCTP (3000 Ci/mmol)	2 µL
Klenow polymerase (5 U/µL)	2 µL
Total	150 µL

3. 10 min incubation at 20°C.
4. Removal of free nucleotides by two precipitations with ammonium acetate 2M-ethanol.
5. Electrophorese through a 2% agarose gel in Tris acetate EDTA buffer.
6. Vacuum dry the gel and radioautography.

4. *In Situ* Detection of Apoptotic Nuclei

The principle of the method is to reveal, within tissue sections, nuclei containing high densities of DNA ends. To this end, the enzymatic DNA end-labeling method has been transposed onto thin sections of paraffin-embedded prefixed mammalian organs (Gavrieli et al., 1992). The major advantage of this histological approach over global DNA extraction from tissues is to identify the nature and localization of apoptotic cells with the resolution of light microscopy. The major limitation of this method is that the DNA fragmentation phase is transient at the level of individual cells (Gavrieli et al., 1992). Hence, the probability of observing nuclei containing fragmented DNA in tissue sections is stringently dependent on the proportion and distribution of cells committed to apoptosis, both in time and space. This may explain why apoptotic nuclei cannot be detected through such techniques in slow neurodegenerative diseases (Migheli et al., 1994). For the purpose of *in situ* assessment of apoptosis, it should be stressed, however, that DNA laddering *per se* has been found less transient (1–3 h) than morphological hallmarks like apoptotic bodies or nucleic shrinkage (a few minutes), as followed on leukocyte apoptosis in vitro (Gavrieli et al., 1992).

A second possible limitation is that, in fact, some DNA breaks are not specific for apoptotic cells. They are also present in other biological situations, as in dividing cells at the level of replication forks, or in quiescent cells after genotoxic treatments (Maehara et al., 1989, 1990), perhaps in relation to intense DNA repair activity. More annoying, numerous DNA breaks occur randomly in necrotic cells, as in tissues dissected from animals not soon enough after death. However, apoptosis-associated DNA breaks should most often be discriminated from other situations of DNA fragmentation. Indeed, necrotic DNA fragmentations should appear more widespread than apoptotic ones (Migheli et al., 1994) and, in turn, DNA ends caused by DNA recombination or replication processes are expected to be much less abundant than in apoptotic cells.

Theoretically, most techniques described above for labeling DNA ends are adaptable to histological sections. Originally, DNA ends were revealed *in situ* by a nick-translation procedure, using the *E. coli* DNA polymerase I (Anai et al., 1988). More recently, the same enzyme has also been used successfully for detecting apoptotic cells (Gold et al., 1993;

Wijsman et al., 1993; Norman et al., 1995). A possible improvement of the labeling method can be provided by a two-step labeling procedure (Wood et al., 1993) using a DNA polymerase with high 3' → 5' exonuclease activity, such as the native T4 or T7 polymerases. In a first step, the enzyme is incubated with DNA in the absence of nucleotides, thus creating very long protruding 5' ends. In a second step, the recessed 3' ends are filled in by the same enzyme in the presence of the four nucleotides, including radiolabeled ones. This method allows incorporation of a larger number of radioelements into each DNA fragment. Like nick translation, however, this highly sensitive method risks revealing DNA nicks unrelated to apoptosis, thus creating an elevated background of nuclear staining. Another possible bias of this method is that the numerous nicks present in apoptotic DNA (Peitsch et al., 1993a) can impede the recessing activity of the enzyme, and shorten DNA fragments. For this reason, this method should be avoided for end labeling DNA ladders.

A protocol for *in situ* detection of apoptotic nuclei by DNA end labeling with a biotinylated nucleotide in the presence of TdT (TUNEL method, modified from Gavrieli et al., 1992) is detailed in Table 3. The method was initially applied to sections from tissues that had been fixed as a whole with a mixture of 4% paraformaldehyde in 0.1M phosphate buffered saline, dehydrated in graded ethanols (70%, 90%, 95%, 100%, 12 h at least each), defatted overnight in xylene, incubated 12 h in liquid paraffin at 56°C, and embedded in paraffin for regular microtome sectioning. However, this method can be applied equally well, or even better, on cryostat sections of unfixed tissues which have been snapfrozen by immersion in liquid isopentane at −45°C immediately after animal sacrifice, without prefixation. Provided that slide-mounted sections of frozen tissues were fixed at first by immersion in 4% paraformaldehyde solution (in 0.1M PBS), the sensitivity of the method was found to be improved. It must be stressed, however, that histological preservation is poorer than with tissue prefixation. In addition, TUNEL labeling was found to be largely prevented by tissue pretreat-

Table 3
Procedure for Apoptosis Detection *In Situ* Using TdT

Preparation of tissue sections

1. Tissue prefixation: This step can be ommitted.
2. Organ freezing by immersion 20 s in isopentane at –45°C; after 10–15 min drying at –80°C, the sample is wrapped up and kept at –80°C until sectioning.
3. Cryostat sectioning at 10-μm thickness, at –18/–20°C for unfixed tissue or –25/–28°C for prefixed tissue.
4. Collection of tissue sections on precoated slides (*see* Table 4 for poly-L-lysine precoating, and text).

Labeling reaction

1. Fixation of slide-mounted tissue sections by immersion 30 min in a 4% paraformaldehyde solution in 0.1M, pH 7.4 phosphate-buffered saline (PBS) at 4°C. This step must be omitted in cases of sections of prefixed tissue.
2. Rinsing in 0.1M PBS at room temperature.
3. Incubation 15 min at room temperature in a solution of proteinase K (from Tritirachium album, Boehringer, Mannheim, Germany) at 20 μg/mL in 0.1M PBS.
4. Rinsing in PBS 2 × 5 min.
5. Incubation 5 min at room temperature in a solution of H_2O_2 at 2% in 0.1M PBS for blocking of endogenous peroxydases.
6. Rinsing in 0.1M PBS.
7. Rinsing in "TdT buffer": Tris-HCl 30 mM pH 7.5, containing 140 mM sodium cacodylate and 1 mM cobalt chloride.
8. Incubation 1 h at 37°C with biotinylated d-UTP (6 μL of Boehringer stock solution) and terminal-d-transferase (12 μL of Boehringer stock solution in 1 mL of TdT buffer.
9. Rinsing in TB buffer (300 mM sodium chloride and 30 mM sodium citrate), 15 min at room temperature.
10. Rinsing in 0.1M PBS.

Staining reaction

1. Incubation in a solution of bovine serum albumin at 2% in 0.1M PBS, 10 min at room temperature.
2. Rinsing in 0.1M PBS.
3. Incubation with ABC complex (Vectastain kit, Vector Lab, Burlingame, CA) as indicated in kit notice.
4. Rinsings in 0.1M PBS and in 0.05M Tris-HCl, pH 7.6, at room temperature.
5. Staining reaction with a filtered mixture of 0.05M Tris-HCl, pH 7.6, containing 0.05% diaminobenzidine, 0.03% nickel chloride, 0.6%

(continued)

Table 2 *(continued)*

H_2O_2. Time of reaction should be approx 5 min at room temperature, but must be adjusted empirically; reaction can be slowed down by proceeding on ice. The reaction can be stopped at once by immersion of slides in a bath of 0.05*M* Tris-HCl at 4°C.

6. Dehydration in graded ethanols, defatting in xylene, and coverslipping with Depex or Permount.

---

ment with glutaraldehyde, a commonly used fixative; consequently, whether performed before or after sectioning, tissue fixation for TUNEL assays must be achieved with a mixture totally devoid of glutaraldehyde, which rules out, for instance, the use of Bouin's fixative (unpublished observations).

Sections for the TUNEL assay must be collected on glass slides that have been precoated so as to resist to the multiple incubations involved in the procedure, especially the proteinase K step. The best results were obtained with a protocol involving poly-L-lysine precoating of slides (Table 4). In addition, crumbling of the sections off the slides in the course of TUNEL labeling was prevented by performing all incubations and rinsings in drops of respective solutions deposited onto the section-holding slides, themselves placed horizontally in humid boxes. The minimal volume required for incubating a single section 5-mm wide is 100 µL, provided that the sections had been circumlined as closely as possible with hydrophobic varnish, using, for instance, a DAKO-pen. Replacement of one solution by the next must be performed quickly enough to prevent the section drying out.

The specific reagents for 3' end-labeling, i.e., TdT and biotinylated dUTP, should be more diluted on sections than on purified DNA extracts, in order to minimize background labeling of nonapoptotic nuclei. Dilutions indicated in Table 3 have been optimized for Boehringer products on 10-µm thick sections of freshfrozen olfactory organs from adult mice.

Biotinylated d-UTP bound to tissue sections can thereafter be revealed with avidin-coupled chromogenic systems; the protocol listed in Table 3 was based on ABC-peroxydase Vectastain kit (Vector) using DiAmino-Benzidine as a chromogen.

Table 4
Slide Precoating

1.	Immerse slides overnight in a 0.5% HCl containing ethanol.
2.	Rinse under tap water 2–3 h.
3.	Rinse in distilled water three times.
4.	Dip slide rack for 5 min into a solution of Poly-L-Lysine (Sigma, St. Louis, MO, P1524) at 0.01% in 10 mM Tris-HCl buffer at pH = 8.
5.	Dry at 37°C and store in dust-free box.

5. Application to the Detection of Neuronal Apoptosis in the Olfactory Epithelium of Adult Mice

5.1. The Peripheral Olfactory System of Adult Mammals as a Model of Neuronal Apoptosis

The olfactory neuroepithelium lines up the convolutions of the remote part of the nasal cavity, termed olfactory turbinates. It is composed of three layers:

1. The medial layer is made up predominantly of odorant-receptive sensory neuron perikarya. Each of these neurons possesses a single, unbranched, apical dendrite extending to the epithelial surface, and a basal axon terminating in glomeruli of the olfactory bulb, wherein it impinges synaptically onto dendrites of relay centripetal neurons and of periglomerular interneurons. Olfactory neuron axons are packed into bundles within underlying lamina propria, where they are wrapped up by glial processes of "ensheathing cells"; the axon bundles together constitute the olfactory cranial nerve and enter the cranial cavity through fenestrations in the cribriform plate of the ethmoid bone.
2. The superficial layer contains the dendrites of sensory neurons, terminated by knobs and cilia endowed with receptors for odorant molecules, and intermingled supporting cells, i.e., epithelial cells of unknown function.

3. The basal layer, residing along the basal lamina in the depth of the epithelium, is composed mainly of undifferentiated cells of neural origin that ensure the continuous renewal of sensory neurons, the life span of which is limited to a few weeks in mammals (Graziadei, 1973; Graziadei and Monti-Graziadei, 1978; Moulton, 1974). All through adult life, sensory neurons that die are replaced by the mitotic activity of basal cells; stem cell-derived progenies differentiate into new olfactory neurons and grow centripetal axons that establish synaptic connections in the olfactory bulb (Monti-Graziadei and Graziadei, 1979). This property of the olfactory neuroepithelium, unique in the adult mammalian nervous system, provides it with regenerative capacity, i.e., ability to recover from injury.

The cell dynamics of mammalian olfactory neuroepithelium can be experimentally accelerated and synchronized in vivo, either by removal of the olfactory bulb, i.e., the unique synaptic target of mature sensory neurons (bulbectomy; Schwartz-Levey et al., 1991), or by sectioning of the olfactory nerve (axotomy; Monti-Graziadei and Graziadei, 1979; Monti-Graziadei et al., 1980). Both types of surgery have long been known to induce a 70% decrease of neuroepithelium thickness, corresponding to the loss of 40–50% of mature sensory neurons, by 4 d postoperative in vivo; this neurodegeneration is followed by a massive and transient stimulation of mitotic activity of basal stem cells, peaking 4–5 d postlesion in the mouse (Schwartz-Levey et al., 1991); subsequent differentiation of stem neuron progenies progressively leads to neuroepithelium regeneration. In addition, unilateral lesions of either type promote a degeneration/regeneration cycle only on the ipsilateral side of the olfactory organ, because of the lack of any crossed projection within the peripheral olfactory pathway of vertebrates. Therefore, transverse sections of olfactory turbinates from unilaterally lesioned animals provide both targetless and control olfactory epithelia, which is a great facility for histochemical assessments.

The deafferentation-induced sequence of degeneration-regeneration in vertebrate olfactory epithelium has been known for a very long time (LeGros-Clark, 1951). The cytology and biology of neuronal differentiation (Monti-Graziadei and Graziadei, 1979) and, more recently, of stem cell mitoses (Schwartz-Levey et al., 1991) have been well characterized. However, the mechanism and origin of neuron losses had never been investigated in this system.

5.2. Kinetic Analysis of the Apoptotic Response to the Synaptic Ablation

We have investigated the mechanism by which the neuronal population of the sensory epithelium massively degenerates after synaptic target ablation. To this aim, the level of olfactory neuron apoptoses was measured in a course of time following their synaptic target ablation. Olfactory mucosae were dissected from mice that were sacrificed at various intervals, ranging from 1 h to 8 d following bilateral bulbectomy. DNAs were prepared as described in Table 2, in sufficient amounts (250 μg DNA/starting from 35 mg of fresh material) to yield visible precipitates. The precipitates were transferred into new tubes, rinsed with 70% ethanol, and allowed to air dry. After solubilization in H_2O, DNA contents were carefully quantified by UV absorbance, so as to adjust all extracts up to the same DNA concentration. From each preparation, 1 μg was submitted to labeling reactions as indicated in Table 3. One-tenth of the reactions were electrophoresed through a 2% agarose-Tris acetate EDTA gel (Fig. 2). The gel was dried and apposed onto an X-ray film in a light-proof cassette. The intensities of the two nucleosome-sized fragments were monitored on the radioautogram (Fig. 2 bottom) by using the Scan-Analysis program (Biosoft, Cambridge, UK). Radioautographic exposure time had to be selected in order to reveal the differences of ladder intensities. In the present case, very long time exposures clearly revealed the existence of apoptotic fragmentations in control olfactory mucosae (not shown), possibly linked to the background of spontaneous renewing of this neuronal population (Graziadei, 1973; Moulton,

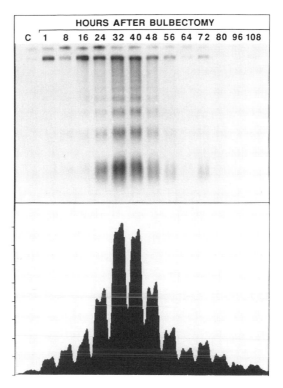

Fig. 2. Evolution of DNA fragmentation in olfactory mucosae. in course of time following bulbectomy. **(Top)** Radioautogram of ^{32}P-labeled DNA ladders obtained as described in Table 2, after electrophoresis through a 2% agarose gel. **(Bottom)** Horizontal scan of the above radioautogram, at the level of the two nucleosome-sized DNA fragments.

1974; Graziadei and Monti-Graziadei, 1978). Interestingly, the increased incorporation of radioactivity into the high molecular weight DNA, at earlier times following bulbectomy (Fig. 2), strongly suggests that the wave of DNA fragmentation is preceded by the accumulation of nicks in DNA, as postulated by the apoptotic DNA fragmentation model (Peitsch et al., 1993a).

5.3. Localization of Apoptotic Cells in Tissue Sections of Olfactory Turbinates

Unilateral olfactory bulbectomy is followed within 2–3 d by a severe involution of ipsilateral olfactory neuroepithe-

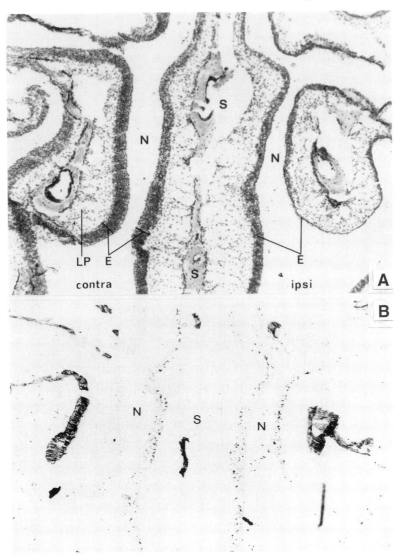

Fig. 3. Accumulation of apoptotic nuclei on the lesioned side of the olfactory mucosa after unilateral olfactory bulbectomy. **(A)** Nissl-stained mouse olfactory turbinates after unilateral olfactory bulbectomy. The striking reduction of neuroepithelium thickness is clearly visible on the side ipsilateral to bulbectomy (right, "ipsi") when compared to the side still connected to olfactory bulb (left, "contra"). This dramatic tissue involution is the consequence of extensive loss of mature olfactory neurons. **(B)** Adjacent section processed by the TUNEL method as described in Table 3.

lium (Fig. 3A). This phenomenon has been reported for a long time as being caused by the selective degeneration of mature sensory neurons of the olfactory mucosa (Monti-Graziadei and Graziadei, 1979; Schwartz-Levey et al., 1991). We applied the TUNEL method, as described above, to cross-sections of olfactory turbinates from mice unilaterally bulbectomized 40–80 h before sacrifice, i.e., at time periods ranging from the peak to the end of DNA laddering activity induced in olfactory mucosa by bulbectomy (Fig. 2). In this material, numerous TUNEL-stained, apoptotic nuclei were detected all along olfactory turbinates ipsilaterally to the bulbectomy, strictly restricted to olfactory epithelium (Fig. 3B). The contralateral neuroepithelium was almost devoid of apoptotic nuclei, except along the nasal septum; this is probably caused by surgical inaccuracy, since olfactory neurons located along the nasal septum project onto the medial aspect of the ipsilateral olfactory bulb (Astic and Saucier, 1986; Saucier and Astic, 1986; Astic et al., 1987). At higher magnification, apoptotic nuclei are found in the inner part of the neuroepithelium (Fig. 4), at the level known to contain the perikarya of mature sensory neurons. It must be noted that, in some instances, Nissl-stained nuclei corresponding to the TUNEL-labeled ones in adjacent sections, appear abnormally dense (Fig. 4), which is caused by the apoptosis-related chromatin compaction and nuclear condensation. This alteration of light microscopic morphology provides the basis for detection of apoptotic nuclei with mere nuclear dyes like Hoechst fluo-

---

Fig. 3 (*continued from previous page*) The apoptotic nuclei appear as dark spots. Labeled nuclei are located only on the bulbectomized side (right) of the olfactory turbinates, except along nasal septum both sides of which are equally enriched in apoptotic nuclei. Since olfactory neurons lining the nasal septum are known to project onto the medialmost part of the olfactory bulbs, these apoptoses are likely to result from surgical inaccuracies on unilaterally bulbectomizing. Abbreviations: E, olfactory neuroepithelium; LP, lamina propria; N, nasal cavity; S, nasal septum; ipsi, ipsilateral to bulbectomy; contra, contralateral to bulbectomy.

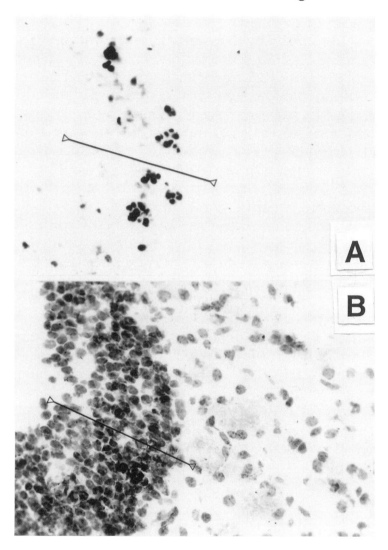

Fig. 4. Localization of apoptotic nuclei at the level of the olfactory neuronal cell body layer. **(A)** High magnification of TUNEL-labeled section of olfactory turbinates ipsilateral to bulbectomy. Apoptotic nuclei are clearly visible as sharply dense masses within the tissue lining the nasal cavity; which observation of the same area of the Nissl-stained adjacent section (*see* **[B]**) permits identification as the inner part of the olfactory neuroepithelium, at the level of the neuron cell body layer. (B) Nissl-stained section of olfactory turbinates, adjacent to that shown in (A) Olfactory mucosa appear composed of two main layers: the neuroepithelium, which contains a higher density of cell bodies, including those of olfatory neurons;

rescent dye or toluidine blue (Pellier and Astic, 1994). In the present case, TUNEL assay allowed us to demonstrate that bulbectomy-induced thinning of olfactory epithelium is definitely caused by apoptotic elimination of mature olfactory neurons, and strongly suggests that the synaptic target of these neurons produces a signal that tonically inhibits triggering of an apoptosis program. In addition, TUNEL-labeled nuclei were frequently observed in clusters, as already reported in other tissues (Gavrieli et al., 1992; Migheli et al., 1994).

Curiously, the number of apoptotic nuclei detected by the TUNEL assay on similar series of regularly spaced olfactory turbinate sections was not much different in mice sacrificed at different times post-bulbectomy. Quantification of TUNEL-stained sections thus failed to reveal the kinetics that had been clearly observed on crude mucosal DNA extracts from bilaterally bulbectomized mice (Michel et al., 1994). This observation, along with similar recent other ones (Rouiller et al., 1995), suggest that TUNEL assays should be used only for qualitative purposes.

Acknowledgments

We thank Veronique Pellier for her advice and help in optimizing the *in situ* labeling of apoptotic nuclei in olfactory mucosa. This work was supported by the "Association pour la Recherche sur le Cancer."

Fig. 4 *(continued from previous page)* and the underlying lamina propria, consisting of connective tissue, bundles of axons of the olfactory neurons and glial cells. On both (A) and (B) figures, the bar between the two hollow triangles indicates the extent of neuroepithelium; nasal cavity is located top left. Apoptotic nuclei are obviously clustered, suggesting that the induction of neuron apoptosis could be triggered synchronously at the level of some sensory units. Some clusters of TUNEL-stained nuclei (A) can be detected also on the ajacent section (B) as abnormally stained by cresyl-violet. This more intense staining reveals the cellular shrinking which occurs during apoptosis.

References

Anai H., Maehara Y., and Sugimachi K. (1988) *In situ* nick translation method reveals DNA strand scission in HeLa cells following heat treatment. *Cancer Lett.* **40,** 33–38.

Appleby D. W. and Modak S. P. (1977) DNA degradtion in terminally differentiating lens fiber cells from chick embryos. *Proc. Natl. Acad. Sci. USA* **74,** 5579–5583.

Astic L. and Saucier D. (1986) Anatomical mapping of the neuroepithelial projection to the olfactory bulb in the rat. *Brain Res. Bull.* **16,** 445–454.

Astic L., Saucier D., and Holley A. (1987) Topographical relationships between olfactory receptor cells and glomerular foci in the rat olfactory bulb. *Brain Res.* **424,** 144–152.

Ausubel F. M., Brent R., Kingston R. E., Moore D. D., Seidman J. G., Smith J. A., and Struhl K., eds. (1994) *Current Protocols in Molecular Biology,* vol. 1, section 2.2., Wiley, New York.

Brune B., Hartzell P., Mcotera P., and Orrenius S. (1991) Spermine prevents endonuclease activation and apoptosis in thymocytes. *Exp. Cell Res.* **195,** 323–329.

Brush W., Kleine L., and Tenniswood M. (1990) The biochemistry of cell death by apoptosis. *Biochem. Cell. Biol.* **88,** 1071–1074.

Ellis R. E., Yuan J., and Horvitz H. R. (1991) Mechanisms and functions of cell death. *Annu. Rev. Cell Biol.* **7,** 663–698.

Estus S., Zaks W. J., Freeman R. S., Gruda M., Bravo R., and Johnson J., E. M. (1994) Altered gene expression in neurons during programmed cell death: identification of cjun as necessary for neuronal apoptosis. *J. Cell Biol.* **127,** 1717–1727.

Filipkowski R. K., Hetman M., Kaminska B., and Kaczmarek L. (1994) DNA fragmentation in rat brain after intraperitoneal administration of kainate. *NeuroReport* **5,** 1538–1540.

Forloni G., Angeretti N., Chiesa R., Monzani E., Salmona M., Bugiani O., and Tagliavini F. (1993) Neurotoxicity of a prion protein fragment. *Nature* **362,** 543–546.

Freeman R. S., Estus S., and Johnson J., E.M. (1994) Analysis of cell cycle-related gene expression on postmitotic neurons: selective induction of *cyclin D1* during programmed cell death. *Neuron* **12,** 343–355.

Gavrieli Y., Sherman Y., and Ben-Sasson S. A. (1992) Identification of programmed cell death *in situ* via specific labeling of nuclear DNA fragmentation. *J. Cell Biol.* **119,** 493–501.

Gold R., Schmied M., Rothe G., Zischler H., Breitschopf H., Wekerle H., and Lassman H. (1993) Detection of DNA fragmentation in apoptosis: application of *in situ* nick translation to cell culture systems and tissue sections. *J. Histochem. Cytochem.* **41,** 1023–1030.

Graziadei P. P. C. (1973) Cell dynamics in the olfactory mucosa. *Tissue Cell* **5,** 113–131.

Graziadei P. P. C. and Monti-Graziadei A. G. (1978) Continuous nerve cell renewal in the olfactory system, in *Development of Sensory Systems*. Jacobson M., ed., Springer, Berlin.

Greenlund L. J. S., Deckwerth T. L., and Johnson J. E. M. (1995) Superoxyde dismutase delays neuronal apoptosis, A role for reactive oxygen species in programmes neuronal death. *Neuron* **14**, 303–315.

Hirt B. (1967) Selective extraction of polyoma DNA from infected mouse cell cultures. *J. Mol. Biol.* **26**, 365–369.

Joseph R., Li W., and Han E. (1993) Neuronal death cytoplasmic calcium and internucleosomal DNA fragmentation: evidence for DNA fragments being released from cells. *Mol. Brain Res.* **17**, 70–76.

Kerr J. F. R., Searle J., Harmon B. V., and Bishop C. J. (1987) Apoptosis, in *Perspectives on Mammalian Cell Death*. Potten C. S., ed., Oxford University Press, Oxford, pp. 93–128.

Kerr J. F. R., Willie A. H., and Currie A. R. (1972) Apoptosis: a basic phenomenon with wide-ranging implications in tissue kinetics. *Br. J. Cancer* **26**, 239–257.

Kure S., Tominaga T., Yoshimoto T., Tada K., and Narisawa K. (1991) Glutamate triggers internucleosomal DNA cleavage in neuronal cells. *Biochem. Biophys. Res. Commun.* **179**, 39–45.

LeGros-Clark W. E. (1951) The projection of the olfactory epithelium on the olfactory bulb in the rabbit. *J. Neurol.* Psychiatry **14**, 1–10.

Lockshin R. A. and William C. M. (1965) Programmed cell death. 1. Cytology of degeneration in the intersegmental muscles of the pernyi silkmoth. *J. Insect Physiol.* **11**, 1231–1233.

Loo D. T., Copani A., Pike C. J., Whittemore E. R., Walencewicz A. J., and Cotman C. W. (1993) Apoptosis is induced beta-amyloid in cultured central nervous system neurons. *Proc. Natl. Acad. Sci. USA* **90**, 7951–7955.

MacManus J. P., Buchan A. M., Hil I. E., Rasquinha I., and Preston E. (1993) Global ischemia can cause DNA fragmentation indicative of apoptosis in rat brain. *Neurosci. Lett.* **164**, 89–92.

Maehara Y., Anai H., Kusumoto T., Sakaguchi Y., and Sugimachi K. (1989) Nick translation detection *in situ* of cellular DNA strand break induced by radiation. *Am. J. Pathol.* **134**, 7–10.

Maehara Y., Anai H., Sakaguchi Y., Kusumoto T., Emi Y., and Sugimachi K. (1990) Detection of DNA strnd breaks in HeLa cells in vitro and in mouse sarcoma 180 cells in vivo induced by an alkylating agent carboquone using *in situ* nick translation. *Oncology* **47**, 282–286.

Michel D., Moyse E., Brun G., and Jourdan F. (1994) Induction of apoptosis by synaptic target ablation in rat olfactory neuroepithelium. *NeuroReport* **5**, 1329–1332.

Migheli A., Cavalla P., Marino S., and Schiffer D. (1994) A study of apoptosis in normal and pathologic nervous tissue after *in situ* end-labeling of DNA strand breaks. *J. Neurophat. Exp. Neurol.* **53**, 606–616.

Monti-Graziadei A. G. and Graziadei P. P. C. (1979) Studies on neuronal plasticity and regeneration in the olfactory system, morphologic and functional characteristics of the olfactory sensory neuron, in *Neural Growth and Differenciation.* Meisami E. and Brazier M. A. B., eds., Raven, New York, pp. 373–396.

Monti-Graziadei A. G., Karlan M. S., Bernstein J. J., and Graziadei P. P. C. (1980) Reinnervation of the olfactory bulb after section of the olfactory nerve in monkey. *Brain Res.* **189,** 343–354

Moulton D. G. (1974) Dynamics of cell populations in the olfactory epithelium. *Ann. NY Acad. Sci.* **237,** 52–61.

Norman D. J., Feng L., Cheng S. S., Gubbay J., Chan E., and Heintz N. (1995) The lurcher gene induces apoptotic death in cerebellar Purkinje cells. *Development* **121,** 1183–1193.

Peitsch M. C., Muller C., and Tschopp J. (1993a) DNA fragmentation during apoptosis is caused by frequent single-strand cuts. *Nucleic Acids Res.* **21,** 4206–4209.

Peitsch M. C., Polzar B., Stephan H., Crompton T., Robson MacDonald H., Mannherz H. G., and Tschopp J. (1993b) Characterization of the endogenous deoxyribonuclease involved in nuclear DNA fragmentation during apoptosis (programmed cell death). *EMBO J.* **12,** 371–377.

Pellier V. and Astic L. (1994) Cell death in the developing olfactory epithelium of rat embryos. *Dev. Brain Res.* **79,** 307–315.

Rosl F. (1992) A simple and rapid method for detection of apoptosis in human cells. *Nucleic Acids Res.* **20,** 5243.

Rouiller D., Didier A., Coronas V., Moyse E., Jourdan F., and Droy-Lefaix M. T. (1995) Effet de l'extrait de Ginkgo biloba sur l'apoptose des neurones olfactifs primaires induite par axotomie. In 2eme Colloque de la Societe Francaize des Neurosciences. Lyon France, pp. 84.

Sambrook J., Fritsch E. F., and Maniatis T. (1989) *Molecular Cloning: A Laboratory Manual.* Cold Spring Harbor Laboratory Press, Cold Spring Harbor, NY.

Saucier D. and Astic L. (1986) Analysis of the topographical organization of olfactory epithelium projections in the rat. *Brain Res. Bull.* **16,** 455–462.

Schwartz L. M. (1991) The role of cell death genes during development. *Bioessays* **13,** 389–395.

Schwartz L. M., Smith S. W., Jones M. E. E., and Osborne B. A. (1993) Do all programmed cell deaths occur via apoptosis? *Proc. Natl. Acad. Sci. USA* **90,** 980–984.

Schwartz-Levey M., Chikaraishi D. M., and Kauer J. S. (1991) Characterization of potential precursor populations in the mouse olfactory epithelium using immunocytochemistry and autoradiography. *J. Neurosci.* **11,** 3556–3564.

Smeyne R. J., Vendrell M., Hayward M., Baker S. J., Miao G. G., Schilling K., Robertson L. M., Curran T., and Morgan J. I. (1993) Continuous *c-fos* expression precedes programmed cell death *in vivo*. *Nature* **363,** 166–169.

Tilly J. L. and Hsueh A. J. W. (1993) Microscale autoradiographic method for the qualitative and quantitative analysis of apoptotic DNA fragmentation. *J. Cell. Physiol.* **154,** 519–526.

Tomei L. D., Shapiro J. P., and Cope F. O. (1993) Apoptosis in C3H/10$_{1/2}$ mouse embryonic cells: evidence for internucleosomal DNA modification in the absence of double-strand cleavage. *Proc. Natl. Acad. Sci. USA* **90,** 853–857.

Ucker D., Obermiller P. S., Eckhart W., Apgar J. R., Berger N. A., and Meyers J. (1992) Genome digestion is a dispensable consequence of physiological cell death mediated by cytotoxic T lymphocytes. *Mol. Cell. Biol.* **12,** 3060–3069.

Wijsman J. H., Honker R. R., Keijzer R., van de Velde C. J. H., Cornelisse C. J., and van Dierendonck J. H. (1993) A new method to detect apoptosis in paraffin sections: *in situ* end-labeling of fragmented DNA. *J. Histochem. Cytochem.* **41,** 7–12.

Wood K. A., Dipascale B., and Youle R. J. (1993) *In situ* labeling of granula cells for apoptosis–associated DNA fragmentation reveals different mechanisms of cell loss in developing cerebellum. *Neuron* **11,** 621–632.

Wyllie A. H. (1980) Glucocorticoid-induced thymocyte apoptosis is associated with endogenous endonuclease activation. *Nature* 555,556.

Wyllie A. H., Kerr J. F. R., and Currie A. R. (1980) Cell death: the significance of apoptosis. *Int. Rev. Cytol.* **68,** 251–306.

Both Irreversible Neuronal Death and Reversible Neuronal Stress Are Associated with Increased Levels of Statin, a Marker of Cell Cycle Arrest

Patricia Boksa, Uwe Beffert, Doris Dea,
Richard Alonso, Dayan O'Donnell,
and Judes Poirier

1. Introduction

It is well known that cell death forms an important part of normal developmental and plastic processes in the brain. For example, during development, proliferating neuronal precursors generate a population of differentiated neurons, some of which make contact with their targets and survive. Neurons that cannot make appropriate targets activate an endogenous gene-directed death program (Cunningham, 1982; Oppenheimer, 1991). Thus, there is an important relationship between cell proliferation, differentiation, and death in neurons.

One of the first signals that can be detected in cells entering a phase of proliferation is the induction of primary response genes including c-fos, c-myc, c-jun, ras, and the heat-shock protein 70 (HS70) (Nishikura and Murray, 1987; Kovary and Bravo, 1991; Trump and Berezesky, 1992; Whitfield, 1992). However a currently puzzling observation in cell biology is the fact that cell injury and programmed cell death also activate these same primary response genes.

From: *Neuromethods, Vol. 29: Apoptosis Techniques and Protocols*
Ed: J. Poirier Humana Press Inc.

Thus it appears that, in some tissues, cells destined to die via apoptosis transiently but abortively re-enter the cell cycle, before proceeding onto death (*see* Wang et al., 1994). For example, in the involuting ventral prostate, cells undergoing programmed cell death show not only an induction of proliferation-related c-fos, c-myc, ras, and the heat-shock protein 70 (Buttyan et al., 1988), but also induction of p53 (Zhang et al., 1994), a suppressor protein known to block the cell cycle. A similar upregulation of expression of c-fos, c-myc, c-jun, and cd2, as well as bromodeoxyuridine labeling indicative of DNA synthesis, has been reported to occur in dying 3T3 fibroblasts (Wang et al., 1994). The presence of p53 has also been associated with programmed cell death in murine and human cell lines (Yonish-Rouach et al., 1991; Shaw et al., 1992) and in another nontransformed nonneuronal tissue undergoing active apoptosis, i.e., irradiated thymocytes (Clarke et al., 1993; Lowe et al., 1993).

The cascade of molecular events leading to cell death in various nonneuronal cells offers some intriguing homologies with neuronal injury caused by excitotoxicity or deafferentation. Following neuronal insult or selective deafferentation, neurons in rodent brain have been shown to synthesize high levels of proteins encoded by primary response genes including c-fos, c-myc, c-jun, jun-b, jun-d, and heat-shock protein 70 (Leah et al., 1991; Chen and Hillman, 1992; Dragunow, 1992; Kawagoe et al., 1992; Nitsch and Frotscher, 1992; Sloviter and Lowenstein, 1992; Kenward et al., 1994). C-fos has also recently been shown to be overexpressed in the hippocampus of human subjects with Alzheimer's disease (AD), in selectively vulnerable areas such as the CA 1 (Zhang et al., 1992). Recently, Sakhi et al. (1994) have demonstrated increased levels of p53 mRNA in brain regions exhibiting morphological and DNA damage following systemic administration of kainate, whereas Chopp et al. (1992) have demonstrated a diffuse immunostaining for p53 in necrotic brain areas following middle cerebral artery occlusion in the rat. Thus, these studies demonstrate that irreversible injury to neuronal tissue can be associated with induction of both proliferation-related gene products and also with a protein that suppresses the cell cycle. An important question that remains, however, is whether induction of antiproliferative genes such as p53 in terminally differentiated neurons is necessarily associated with *irreversible* commitment to cell death. Alternatively, may induction of such genes also be associated with early and reversible (i.e., nonlethal) neuronal perturbation?

The main aim of the present study was to address this question. For this, we examined expression of a marker of cell cycle arrest in models of CNS damage in which there is either clear neuronal death or only sublethal neuronal injury. The marker of cell cycle arrest chosen was statin. Statin is a 57-kDa nuclear protein demonstrated to be uniquely associated with the Go (quiescent, nonproliferating) state in a wide number of cell types throughout the body, including CNS neurons, astrocytes, fibroblasts, epithelial cells, hepatocytes, pineal cells, and glioma cell lines (Wang, 1985; Bisonnette et al., 1990; Federoff et al., 1990; Schipper and Wang, 1990; Ann et al., 1991; Tsanaclis et al., 1991). In the brain, statin levels are several-fold higher in terminally differentiated neurons than in glia (Schipper and Wang, 1990; Tsanaclis et al., 1991). Recent results indicate that statin coprecipitates with a 45-kDa serine/threonine kinase (Lee et al., 1992). Statin is also associated with a third protein characterized as retinoblastoma (RB) protein in its unphosphorylated form (Wang et al., 1994), the form necessary for the latter protein to be antiproliferatively functional. Several other observations provide further evidence for the specificity of statin expression in the nonproliferative state. For example, statin immunoreactivity in the nucleus disappears when serum-deprived, growth-arrested fibroblasts are allowed to re-enter the cell cycle (Wang and Lin, 1986). Additionally, in transformed cells, detection and quantification of statin has been used to monitor the nonproliferating and/or dying fraction of a tumor population (Schipper et al., 1990).

The present study examined statin in three different in vivo models of hippocampal neuronal damage. Two of these models were the hippocampus of patients with AD and the hippocampus of rats with kainate lesions in CA3, both models in which neuronal cell death clearly occurs (Nadler, 1981; Van Hoesen et al., 1991). The third model was the hippocampus of rats with entorhinal cortex-lesions (ECL). This third model mimics the entorhinal deafferentation of hippocampal targets characteristic of AD, however hippocampal neurons are reported to be spared due to extensive reactive synaptogenesis that takes place in this model (Lynch et al., 1976; Scheff et al., 1980). Thus, these in vivo models represent cases of both lethal and sublethal injury to hippocampal neurons. Finally, an in vitro model of excitotoxic insult to embryonic rat cultured hippocampal neurons was used to examine the early time course of statin expression in comparison to signs of neuronal death as determined by vital staining.

2. Materials and Methods

2.1. Human Brain Tissues

All human brain tissues were obtained from the Douglas Hospital Brain Bank, McGill University, Montreal, Canada. Neuropathological confirmation of AD was performed according to a modification of the methods described by Khachaturian (1985). The protocol is based on age-related, neocortical and hippocampal plaque scores combined with a clinical history of dementia. Brains from five patients with AD and seven with no neurological disease were dissected, frozen in isopentane (–40°C) and stored at –80°C. Age, sex, and postmortem intervals were matched.

2.2. Kainate Lesions of Hippocampus in Rats

Adult Sprague-Dawley rats (150–200 g) were anesthetized with pentobarbital (Nembutal: 50 mg/kg, ip) and mounted in a Kopf stereotaxic frame. Animals received unilateral injections of kainic acid (2 μg in 1 μL of saline) into the dorsal hippocampus using a Hamilton microsyringe. The solution was injected over a period of 5 min. Injection coordinates were A:+4.9, L:2.0, V:+1.8. Ten days postsurgery, rats ($n = 3$) were sacrificed by decapitation and brains were prepared for statin immunohistochemistry.

2.3. Entorhinal Cortex-Lesion in Rats

Fisher 344 male rats (375–425 g) received unilateral electrolytic entorhinal cortex-lesions as described previously by Poirier and Nichol (1991). The contralateral side served as an internal control. Sites at nine stereotaxic coordinates per side were lesioned with a 1-mA current of 25 s duration. The electrode was positioned at a 10° angle from the medial to the lateral and the nose bar was lowered to −1.0 mm. The first set of electrolytic lesions was done at 3.3 mm lateral to midline and 0.2 mm posterior to the interaural line. Lesions were made at 2, 4, and 6 mm below the surface of the brain. The electrode was then repositioned at a point 1 mm lateral to the 3.3 mm point and lowered successively to 2, 4, and 6 mm below the surface of the brain. Last, 3 lesions were placed another 0.8 mm lateral and 1.0 mm anterior to the interaural line at 2, 4, and 6 mm from the brain surface. Pilot studies showed that these lesions targeted the medial and lateral entorhinal cortex and part of the parasubiculum. Control animals received either electrical shocks, equivalent in duration to the ECL, at the level of the dura, or a sham operation. After recovery periods of 2, 6, 8, or 30 d, during which there was a mild loss of body weight, animals were sacrificed, and the brains rapidly dissected. For half of the animals ($n = 6$), both hippocampi were dissected out and frozen at −80°C for protein quantification via Western blot analyses, whereas brains from the second set of animals ($n = 6$) were sectioned (15 µm) for immunohistochemistry on a Bright Cryostat. Entorhinal lesions were monitored using cresyl violet stained sections prepared in the horizontal plane through the area lesioned in the posterior portion of the brain.

2.4. Primary Hippocampal Cell Cultures and N-Methyl-D-Aspartate Toxicity

Hippocampi from embryonic Long-Evans rats (18–19 d gestation) were dissected in Hank's balanced salt solution and mechanically dissociated in Ca^{2+}- and Mg^{2+}-free Hank's solution. The cell suspension was centrifuged (500g, 5 min) and the resulting pelleted cells suspended in Dulbecco's modified Eagle's medium (DMEM) containing 10% (v/v) fetal calf serum, 50 U/mL penicillin, and 50 μg/mL streptomycin. Dissociated cells were plated at a density of 1.5 × 10⁵ cells/cm² on poly-D-lysine (25 μg/mL) coated 35-mm tissue culture plates containing 2 mL of DMEM. For immunocytochemistry experiments, cells were plated on poly-D-lysine-coated 18 mm glass or Aclar plastic coverslips. After 24–30 h, culture medium was replaced with 1 mL of serum-free medium containing DMEM and Ham's F-12 (1:1, v/v) with the N_2 additives described by Bottenstein and Sato (1979), in addition to 50 U/mL penicillin, 50 μg/mL streptomycin, and 8 mM glucose. This low volume of medium markedly improved the quality of the cultures obtained. Cultures were maintained at 37°C in 90% air/10% CO_2 in a humidified incubator. After 8 d in culture, immunoreactivity to glial fibrillary acidic protein was detected in only 6–8% of cells, indicating that these cultures contained mainly neurons.

On d 8 in culture, cells were washed twice with 1 mL Mg^{2+}-free Locke's buffer. Cells were then exposed for 10 min to Locke's buffer containing 500 μM N-methyl-D-aspartate (NMDA). After two washes with 1 mL Locke's buffer, culture media were returned to their original dishes and the cells maintained for different time periods as indicated, before immunocytochemical or immunoblot detection of statin or assessment of neuron viability by a fluorescein diacetate/propidium iodide double-labeling technique described by Didier et al. (1990) and Alonso et al. (1994).

2.5. Statin Immunohistochemistry

Statin immunoreactive neurons in brain sections (15 μm) from rat and humans and in primary hippocampal cell cultures were visualized as modified from the methods of Poirier et al. (1991). Frozen brain sections (15 μm) were allowed to thaw for 25 min at room temperature and were then pretreated with peroxide (30 min, 3% H_2O_2) to block endogenous peroxidase activity and rinsed thoroughly with phosphate-buffered saline (PBS, pH 7.4). Cell cultures were gently rinsed with PBS, fixed with methanol:acetone (1:1, v/v) at −20°C for 30 min and air dried for 30 min. Both tissue sections and cell cultures were then processed for statin immunochemistry using the avidin-biotin peroxidase method (ABC Kit, Vector Laboratories, Burlingame, CA). Tissues were first incubated (30 min) with 1% goat serum to block nonspecific IgG binding. Tissues were then incubated overnight at 4°C with a mouse monoclonal primary antibody (S44) against human statin (generous gift from E. Wang, Lady Davis Institute, McGill University, Montreal, Canada) at a dilution of 1:25,000 or 1:5000. The S44 statin antibody was initially raised against senescent human fibroblast cytoskeleton extracts by Wang (1985) and has been used to identify statin, a 57-kDa protein (Bisonnette et al., 1990; Sester et al., 1990) expressed exclusively in nonproliferating cells and terminally differentiated tissues (Bisonnette et al., 1990; Wang, 1985; Wang and Lin, 1986; Wang, 1989). The specificity of S44 as a Go phase marker has been confirmed in a variety of tissues both in vitro and *in situ* (Wang and Kreuger, 1985; Wang and Lin, 1986; Federoff et al., 1990; Schipper and Wang, 1990; Schipper et al., 1990; Ann et al., 1991). After rinsing with PBS, biotinylated secondary antibodies and avidin-complexed horseradish peroxidase were sequentially applied and the reaction visualized by incubation (23°C) with hydrogen peroxide (0.3%) and 3,3'-diaminobenzidine (0.1%). Typically, reaction product precipitated between 5 and 15 min of incubation. The reaction was stopped by immersion of the sections in a PBS bath. Reaction product was not observed in sections incubated with control ascites fluid in place of the S44 antibody.

2.6. Western Blot Analysis of Statin Levels

The content of statin in rat hippocampus was determined by Western blot analysis as modified from Poirier et al. (1993). For whole hippocampal tissue, an aliquot of hippocampal homogenate containing 50 μg of protein was loaded onto a 25-cm, SDS polyacrylamide gel (10%) and run for 3 h at 23°C. For hippocampal cell cultures, 10 μg of protein was solubilized in SDS-PAGE sample buffer (Laemmli, 1970), boiled for 1 min and electrophoresed into an 8% minipolyacrylamide gel. Proteins were transferred to nitrocellulose filters in a Bio-Rad (Richmond, CA) Trans-blot cell and incubated in blocking buffer (5% dried milk, 0.1% Tween-20, 140 mM NaCl, 20 mM Tris-HCl, pH 7.4), followed by a 1 h incubation with a MAb against human statin (S-44), that crossreacts with the rat antigen (dilution 1:2000 or 1:5000). In all Western experiments, alpha-tubulin antibody (Amersham, Oakville, ON, Canada, Cat. # 234-12) was used to detect a protein whose levels did not change. Molecular weight markers (Rainbow Markers, Amersham) were run in adjacent wells. Visualization of bands was done with a chemiluminescence detection kit (RPN 2100, Amersham). Quantification of autoradiographic bands was performed using an MCID image analysis system (St. Catharines, Ontario) equipped for 1D gel analysis. Protein content of homogenates was determined by the microbicinchoninic acid method (Smith et al., 1985). Samples were run in duplicate and individual Western blot experiments were repeated three times.

3. Results

3.1. Regional Distribution of Statin in the Hippocampus of Alzheimer's Disease Subjects

Regional analysis of statin immunoreactivity in human hippocampus was assessed in frozen hippocampal brain sections from control (n = 7) and AD (n = 5) subjects (Fig. 1A). Statin immunoreactivity was markedly increased in CA1 neurons from AD hippocampus compared to control. By contrast, dentate granule cell neurons from AD subjects showed a distribution of statin immunoreactivity similar to that seen in control individuals and the proportion of dentate granule cells that showed high levels of statin immunoreactivity was not significantly different in AD and control individuals. Levels of statin immunoreactivity were also similar in the CA3 region of AD and control subjects.

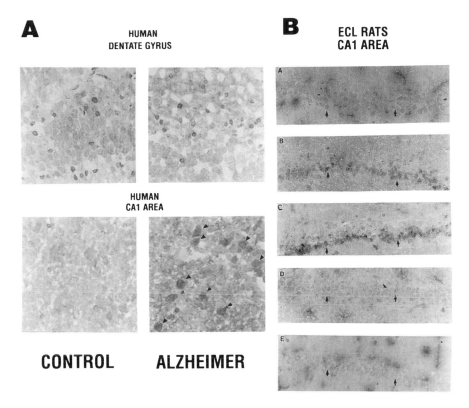

A HUMAN DENTATE GYRUS

B ECL RATS CA1 AREA

HUMAN CA1 AREA

CONTROL **ALZHEIMER**

Fig. 1. Statin immunoreactivity in areas of the hippocampus taken from humans with Alzheimer's disease **(A)** and from rats with entorhinal cortex-lesions **(B)**. (A) Fifteen-micron frozen brain sections from human hippocampus with and without Alzheimer's disease were stained with an MAb to statin (clone S-44, dilution 1:5000), magnification 800×. Age, sex, and postmortem delays were matched. Arrowheads indicate cells showing intense statin immunoreactivity. (B) Fifteen-micron frozen brain sections from rats with and without unilateral entorhinal cortex-lesions were immunostained for statin (antibody S-44, dilution 1:25,000). Photomicrographs (A) through (E) represent pyramidal cell layers of the CA1 region ipsilateral to the lesion from a control (A) and from an entorhinal cortex-lesioned animal at 2 (B), 6 (C), 8 (D), or 30 (E) d postlesion, magnification 200×. Arrows indicate the CA1 pyramidal cell layer. Only background staining could be detected when control hybridoma ascites fluid was substituted for S-44.

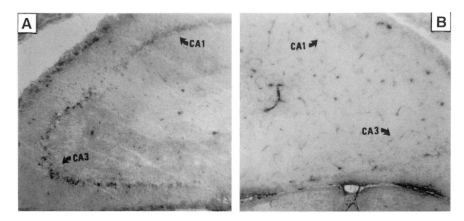

Fig. 2. Statin immunoreactivity in the hippocampus of rats following kainate injections into the dorsal hippocampus. Fifteen micron frozen brain sections from rats with (A) and without (B) unilateral kainate injections into dorsal hippocampus were immunostained for statin (antibody S-44, dilution 1:25,000), magnification 200×. Arrows indicate the locations of the CA1 and CA3 pyramidal cell layers.

3.2. Regional Statin Distribution in the Hippocampus of Kainate-Lesioned Rats

In order to test whether statin is altered in an animal model of acute hippocampal neuron degeneration, statin distribution was assessed in the hippocampus of rats that had received kainate injections into the hippocampus 10 d prior to sacrifice (Fig. 2). Statin immunoreactivity was markedly increased in CA3 hippocampal neurons from kainate-lesioned animals in comparison to controls; a modest elevation of statin immunoreactivity was also observed in the CA1 region from kainate-lesioned animals.

3.3. Statin Levels and Regional Statin Distribution in the Hippocampus of ECL Rats

In order to test whether statin levels are altered following a reportedly nonlethal perturbation of hippocampal neurons, statin levels and distribution were assessed in the hippocampus of rats that had received electrolytic lesions of

ECL RATS
HIPPOCAMPUS

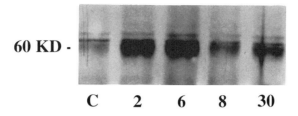

60 KD -

C   2   6   8   30

Fig. 3. Immunoblot detection of statin-related polypeptides in hippo-campal homogenates from entorhinal cortex-lesioned (ECL) rats. Proteins from total hippocampal homogenates were separated by SDS-polyacry-lamide gel electrophoresis and analyzed by Western blotting with an MAb to statin (antibody S-44, dilution 1:5,000). Autoradiogram represents the time course of changes in a 60-kD statin-related peptide in ECL rats (C: control; 2, 6, 8, and 30 d postlesion).

the entorhinal projection to the hippocampus. Western blot analyses of statin levels in total hippocampal homogenates from both control and ECL rats revealed a major band at approx 60 kDa. At 2 d following entorhinal cortex-lesion, the 60-kDa signal in the hippocampus increased by twofold (mean increase from three experiments), compared to basal control levels ($p < 0.05$, Fig. 3). The increase in statin levels was maintained at 6 d postlesion at 2.4 times control levels (mean increase from three experiments, $p < 0.05$). By 8 d postlesion, statin levels were nearly back to control levels, yet still significantly different from control; and by 30 d postlesion, statin levels were no longer significantly elevated.

Immunohistochemical detection of statin revealed a pro-nounced but restricted increase in statin immunoreactivity in pyramidal neurons of the CA1 region at 2 and 6 d post-lesion in ECL rats (Fig. 1B). This increase was no longer observed at 8 or 30 d postlesion. The close correlation over time between changes in statin levels as analyzed by West-ern blot and changes in intensity of immunohistochemical staining in the CA1 following ECL strongly suggests that the

Table 1
Neuronal Cell Counts
in the Hippocampus of Entorhinal Cortex-Lesioned Rats

	Control	Time postlesion (d)			
		2	6	8	30
Brain region					
CA1 area	95 ± 3	98 ± 9	102 ± 15	97 ± 7	108 ± 9
Dentate gyrus	238 ± 17	217 ± 29	224 ± 28	241 ± 27	215 ± 26

Cresyl violet stained sections were used to estimate cell number in the CA1 and dentate granule cell layers of the hippocampus of control rats and of entorhinal cortex-lesioned rats at various times postlesion. Two individuals assessed each section by counting cells ipsilateral and contralateral to the lesion independently and in a double-blind manner. Data are expressed as cell number ± SEM/field ipsilateral to the lesion.

increase in immunohistochemical staining reflects an increase in statin levels. In contrast to the CA1 region, dentate granule cells, which receive most of the entorhinal input to the hippocampus, did not show any alteration in statin immunoreactivity (data not shown). Cell number in the CA1 and dentate gyrus areas remained unchanged during the 2–30 d postlesion period (Table 1). Other brain regions examined (e.g., hypothalamus, temporal and piriform cortices, and ventricular areas) failed to show any alteration in statin expression.

3.4. Statin Expression During NMDA Toxicity in Primary Hippocampal Neuronal Cultures

In order to further characterize the temporal relationship between statin induction and neuronal cell injury, statin expression was monitored in hippocampal cell cultures exposed to lethal concentrations of the excitotoxin, NMDA (Choi et al., 1988). The time course analysis of the effect of NMDA on hippocampal cell cultures indicates that statin expression increased as early as 20 min after a brief exposure to NMDA (Fig. 4A). Parallel experiments on sister cultures indicated no signs of significant cell death, as assessed by vital staining, at 20, 60, or 90 min after NMDA exposure (*see* Alonso et al., 1994). One hundred and fifty minutes after

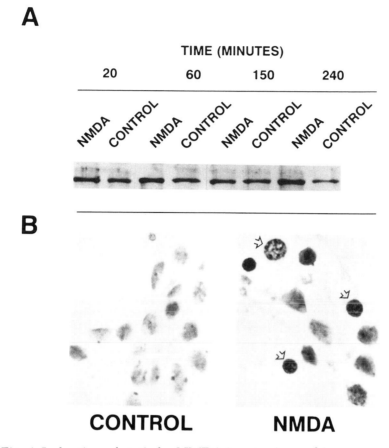

Fig. 4. Induction of statin by NMDA in rat primary hippocampal cell cultures. Serum free primary hippocampal cell cultures were exposed to 500 μ*M* NMDA in Locke's buffer for 10 min, washed, and returned to their original medium for different time periods. **(A)** Proteins (10 μg) harvested at various time points after NMDA exposure were subjected to Western blot immunodetection for statin. Control cultures were exposed to the same buffers in the absence of NMDA. These neuron-enriched (approx 92%) cell cultures showed a single statin band at around 60 kDa. **(B)** Immunocytochemical detection of statin-related polypeptides was performed in sister cultures fixed in acetone-methanol 60 min after NMDA treatment. Magnification 1200×.

NMDA exposure, a very mild cell loss (~10%) was detected, whereas statin levels remained elevated. In contrast, immunocytochemical detection of statin in sister cultures taken 60 min following NMDA treatment, showed that in more than 50% of the neurons exposed to NMDA, statin became progressively associated with the chromatin and underwent marked condensation (Fig. 4B). Twenty-four hours after NMDA exposure, more than 75% of the neurons were dead whereas statin levels remained within control range.

4. Discussion

These results show that expression of statin, a nuclear marker of cell cycle arrest, is increased in four distinct models of hippocampal neuronal distress and/or degeneration. This increase in statin occurs in adult neurons which are terminally differentiated cells, unable to reenter the cell cycle, and thus, already constitutively express high levels of statin. Statin upregulation has previously been associated with the loss of proliferative activity in cell types capable of cycling (Wang, 1985; Wang and Lain, 1986; Fedoroff et al., 1990; Tsanaclis et al., 1991). The current studies utilizing models of hippocampal neuron injury have allowed us to extend these findings to demonstrate that upregulation of this protein can also occur in a terminally differentiated, nonproliferating, cell population.

In the hippocampus of human subjects with AD, statin immunoreactivity was markedly increased in the CA1 region, but not in the dentate gyrus, in comparison to levels detected in neurologically normal, age-matched controls. Major targets for pathology in AD are layers II and IV of the entorhinal cortex (Van Hoesen et al., 1991), which project to the subicular cortex and CA1 zone of the hippocampus. Within the hippocampus itself, there is extensive pathological loss of pyramidal neurons in area CA1 (Van Hoesen et al., 1991). However, dentate granule cell neurons undergo entorhinal deafferentation without marked cell loss in AD (Van Hoesen et al., 1991). Thus, enhanced statin immunoreactivity in the hippocampus in AD appears to correlate, to some degree, with regional cell loss.

In the rat, injection of the excitotoxin, kainate, into the hippocampus resulted in extensive cell loss in the CA3 region

(Nadler, 1981; present study). Intrahippocampal kainate also caused a marked increase in statin immunoreactivity in the CA3 and a modest increase in CA1. However, the dentate, which is spared following intrahippocampal kainate, showed no increase in statin beyond control levels. These results indicate that statin immunoreactivity can also be enhanced in vulnerable areas of the hippocampus in response to acute neuronal degeneration in the rodent.

The third set of experiments attempted to determine whether statin levels in the hippocampus are enhanced only in association with cellular death, or whether levels of the protein may be increased by sublethal perturbations of neuronal populations. For this, we used the ECL rat model. The major hippocampal target of entorhinal cortex afferents is the molecular layer of the dentate gyrus, although minor entorhinal inputs to CA1 and CA3 are also present (Matthews et al., 1976a,b). In young rats, lesion of entorhinal cortex afferents results in a rapid reactive synaptogenesis mainly between axon collaterals of the commissural-associational pathway and the denervated hippocampal targets (Lynch et al., 1976; Scheff et al., 1980). As a result, there is no grossly evident cell loss within hippocampal target areas following ECL. In the present study, we confirm, using quantitative cell counting, that there is no significant cell loss in either the dentate gyrus or CA1 at various times up to 30 d following ECL in young rats. Thus, ECL lesion in young rats can be used as a model of deafferentation (a form of cellular stress or perturbation) of the dentate gyrus and CA1, which does not lead to neuronal death in these regions.

Despite the fact that there was no neuronal loss in the hippocampus of ECL rats, a marked increase in hippocampal statin levels, localized almost exclusively to the CA1 area, was observed at 2 and 6 d postlesion. This increase in statin levels was reversible, with levels returning to control values by 30 d postlesion, and was almost certainly neuronal in origin since reactive astrocytes, which proliferate in response to injury, are statin-negative (Federoff et al., 1990). Enhancement of statin levels in the ECL hippocampus in the absence of cell loss and the reversibility of the statin increase indicate that increases in statin levels are not necessarily accompanied by neuronal death and are not secondary to neuronal degeneration. This raises the possibilities that statin is increased as an early component of the molecular cascade leading to cell death, when the degenerative process is still potentially reversible; and/or statin is increased as a component of a compensatory response designed to restore or maintain cellular homeostasis in injured cells.

The pattern of hippocampal statin induction was very similar in human AD and in ECL rats, despite the fact that the CA1 suffers cell loss in the first condition but not in the second. The fact that dentate granule cells, which receive most of the entorhinal input, show no alteration in statin immunoreactivity indicates that deafferentation per se is not sufficient to induce statin expression in vivo. This conclusion is further supported by our recent findings that fimbria fornix transection, which results in marked cholinergic denervation of the CA1 and dentate gyrus, does not alter hippocampal statin immunostaining (Poirier, unpublished observations). It is also noteworthy that the selective increase in statin immunoreactivity in the CA1 area, but not CA3 or the dentate, following ECL parallels the selective vulnerability of the CA1 in other models of hippocampal injury, such as that resulting from hypoxia/ischemia (Schmidt-Kastner and Freund, 1991).

The differential increase in statin in the CA1 vs the dentate gyrus both in human AD and in ECL rats may relate to the excitatory amino acid inputs to these two regions. Glutamate is the main transmitter utilized by perforant path projections to the hippocampus (White et al., 1977; Fonnum, 1984). High levels of N-methyl-D-aspartate (NMDA) and non-NMDA subtypes of excitatory amino-acid receptors are found both in the CA1 and in the dentate molecular layer (Monaghan et al., 1984; Greenamyre et al., 1985; Monaghan and Cotman, 1985; Ulas et al., 1990a,b). However, glutamate transport sites, which serve to terminate actions of released glutamate, are more numerous in the dentate molecular layer compared to CA1. Furthermore, Anderson et al. (1991) have demonstrated that the dentate gyrus, but not the CA1 area, shows a preferential increase in glutamate transport sites after ECL. Thus, the dentate gyrus may function more effectively than does the CA1 in clearing released glutamate, which in the case of ECL may originate from degenerating entorhinal afferent terminals. This differential glutamate transport has been postulated to account, at least in part, for the observation that CA1 pyramidal neurons are more vulnerable to excitotoxic damage than are dentate granule cells.

The findings with primary cultures of hippocampal neurons support the idea that the selective increase in statin immunoreactivity in the CA1 area following ECL may also relate to the degree of excitatory amino-acid input to this area. These experiments showed that excitotoxic concentrations of NMDA produce an increase in statin levels in cultured hippocampal neurons. Furthermore, statin was clearly overexpressed several hours before the first detection of NMDA-induced neuronal death, as assessed by propidium iodide staining. Thus, in agreement with the present in vivo lesion models, studies with hippocampal cultures also suggest that statin overexpression occurs during the early phases of the process of NMDA toxicity and is probably not the result of the degenerative process itself. Statin levels in hippocampal cultures are also markedly increased by a Ca^{2+} ionophore, A23187 (Alonso et al., 1994). In addition, the temporal profile of statin overexpression we found after NMDA exposure (Alonso et al., 1994; present study) parallels the three phases of altered intracellular Ca^{2+} concentrations induced by glutamate toxicity (Randall and Thayer, 1992). Thus cell culture studies suggest that statin induction in vivo may also be mediated by activation of the NMDA receptor and its associated Ca^{2+} channel.

The selective increase in statin, a marker for cell cycle arrest, in CA1 neurons in the present study parallels induction of the proto-oncogene, c-fos, in the hippocampus of ECL rats (Nitsch and Frotscher, 1992) and of AD subjects (Zhang et al., 1992). In addition, we have recently found, using Western blot analyses, that NMDA-treated hippocampal cultures simultaneously overexpress both statin and c-fos (Poirier, unpublished observations). Thus, in models of both reversible neuronal distress and irreversible neuronal death, there is coordinate induction of proteins involved in both the activation and arrest of the cell cycle in response to cellular injury. It is tempting, although highly speculative, to hypothesize that cell cycle suppressor proteins may act to block the proliferating activity of primary response gene products, yet allow other activities mediated by these gene products, such as those related to growth and differentiation, to function in maintaining or restoring neuronal homeostasis following injury. What is clear is that enhanced expression of statin and of other proteins related to the cell cycle are part of the early response to injury in neurons and other cell types. The precise functional role, if any, of these proteins, either in the degenerative process or in restoration of homeostasis, remains to be determined.

Acknowledgments

We wish to thank Y. Robitaille and R. Quirion from the Douglas Hospital Brain Bank and also Eugenia Wang who provided us with the S-44 (statin) and control antibodies. This work was supported in part by the National Institute on Aging (J. P.; AG 10003), American Alzheimer's Association (J. P.), a career award (J. P.), and a fellowship (R. A.) from the Medical Research Council of Canada.

References

Alonso R., Poirier J., O'Donnell D., Boksa P., and Quirion R. (1994) Statin, a marker of cell cycle arrest, is overexpressed during the early phase of delayed NMDA toxicity in hippocampal cell cultures. *Mol. Cell. Neurosci.* **5,** 530–539.

Anderson K. J., Bridges R. J., and Cotman C. W. (1991) Increased density of excitatory amino acid transport sites in the hippocampal formation following an entorhinal lesion. *Brain Res.* **562,** 285–290.

Ann D. K., Wechsler A., Lin H. H., and Wang E. (1991) Isoproterenol downregulation of statin-related gene expression in the rat parotid gland. *J. Cell Sci.* **100,** 641–647.

Bisonnette R., Lee M. J., and Wang E. (1990) The differentiation process of intestinal epithelial cells is associated with the appearance of statin. *J. Cell Sci.* **95**, 247–254.

Bottenstein R., and Sato G. H. (1979) Growth of a rat neuroblastoma cell line in serum-free supplemented medium. *Proc. Natl. Acad. Sci. USA* **76**, 514–517.

Buttyan R., Zakeri Z., Lockshin R., and Wolgemuth D. (1988) Cascade induction of c-fos, c-myc, and heat-shock 70K transcripts during regression of the ventral prostate gland. *Mol. Endocrinol.* **7**, 650–657.

Chen S. and Hillman D. E. (1992) Transient Fos-expression and dendritic spine plasticity in hippocampal granule cells. *Brain Res.* **577**, 169–174.

Choi D. W., Koh J. Y., and Peters S. (1988) Pharmacology of glutamate neurotoxicity in cortical cell culture. *J. Neurosci.* **8**, 185–196.

Chopp M., Li Y., Zhang Z. G., and Freytag S. O. (1992) p53 expression in brain after middle cerebral artery occlusion in the rat. *Biochem. Biophys. Res. Commun.* **182**, 1201–1207.

Clarke A. R., Purdie C. A., Harrison D. J., Morris R. G., Bird C. C., Hooper M. L., and Wyllie A. H. (1993) Thymocyte apoptosis by p53-dependent and independent pathways. *Nature* **362**, 849–852.

Cunningham T. J. (1982) Naturally-occurring neuron death and its regulation by developing pathways. *Int. Rev. Cytol.* **74**, 163–185.

Didier M., Heaulme P., Soubrie P., Bockaert J., and Pin J. P. (1990) Rapid, sensitive and simple method for quantification of both neurotoxic and neurotrophic effects of NMDA on cultured cerebellar granule cells. *J. Neurosci. Res.* **27**, 25–35.

Dragunow M. (1992) Axotomized medial-diagonal band neurons express Jun immunoreactivity. *Mol. Brain Res.* **15**, 141–144.

Fedoroff S., Ahmed I., and Wang E. (1990) The relationship of expression of statin to the differentiation and cell cycle of astroglia in culture. *J. Neurosci. Res.* **26**, 1–15.

Fonnum F. (1984) Glutamate: a neurotransmitter in mammalian brain. *J. Neurochem.* **42**, 1–11.

Greenamyre J. T., Olson J. M., Penney J., and Young A. B. (1985) Autoradiographic characterization of N-methyl-D-aspartate-, quisqualate- and kainate-sensitive glutamate binding sites. *J. Pharmacol. Exp. Ther.* **233**, 254–263.

Kawagoe J., Abe K., Sato S., Nagano I., Nakamura S., and Kogure K. (1992) Distribution of heat-shock cognate protein (HSC) 70 after transient focal ischemia in rat brain. *Brain Res.* **587**, 195–202.

Kenward N., Hope J., Landon M., and Mayer R. J. (1994) Expression of polyubiquitin and heat-shock protein 70 genes increases in the later stages of disease progression in scrapie-infected mouse brain. *J. Neurochem.* **62**, 1870–1877.

Khachaturian Z. S. (1985) Diagnosis of Alzheimer's disease. *Arch. Neurol.* **42**, 1097–1105.

Kovary K. and Bravo R. (1991) The Jun and Fos protein families are both required for cell cycle progression. *Mol. Cell. Biol.* **11,** 4466–4472.

Laemmli U. K. (1970) Cleavage of structural proteins during the assembly of the head of bacteriophage T4. *Nature* **227,** 680–685.

Leah J. D., Herdegen T., and Bravo R. (1991) Selective expression of Jun protein following axotomy and axonal transport block in peripheral nerves in the rat. *Brain Res.* **566,** 198–207.

Lee M. J., Sandig M., and Wang E. (1992) Statin a protein marker specific for nonproliferating cells is a phosphoprotein and forms an in vivo complex with a 45 kilodalton serine/threonine kinase. *J. Biol. Chem.* **267,** 21,773–21,781.

Lowe S. W., Schmitt E. M., Smith S. W., Osborne B. A., and Jacks T. (1993) p53 is required for radiation-induced apoptosis in mouse thymocytes. *Nature* **362,** 847–849.

Lynch G., Gall C., Rose G., and Cotman C. (1976) Changes in the distribution of the dentate gyrus associational system following unilateral or bilateral entorhinal lesion in the adult brain. *Brain Res.* **110,** 57–71.

Matthews D. A., Cotman C., and Lynch G. (1976a) An electron microscopic study of lesion-induced synaptogenesis in the dentate gyrus of the adult rat. I. Magnitude and time course of degeneration. *Brain Res.* **115,** 1–21.

Matthews D. A., Cotman C., and Lynch G. (1976b) An electron microscopic study of lesion-induced synaptogenesis in the dentate gyrus of the adult rat. II. Reappearance of morphologically normal contacts. *Brain Res.* **115,** 23–41.

Monaghan D. T. and Cotman C. W. (1985) Distribution of N-methyl-D-aspartate-sensitive L-[^{3}H]glutamate binding sites in rat brain. *J. Neurosci.* **5,** 2909–2919.

Monaghan D. T., Yao D., and Cotman C. W. (1984) Distribution of [^{3}H]AMPA binding sites in rat brain as determined by quantitative aultoradiography. *Brain Res.* **324,** 160–164.

Nadler J. V. (1981) Role of excitatory pathways in the hippocampal damage produced by kainic acid. *Adv. Biochem. Psychopharmacol.* **27,** 395–402.

Nishikura K. and Murray J. M. (1987) Antisense DNA of proto-oncogene c-fos blocks renewed growth of quiescent 3T3 cells. *Mol. Cell. Biol.* **7,** 639–649.

Nitsch R. and Frotscher M. (1992) Reduction of post-traumatic transneuronal "early gene" activation and dendritic atrophy by the N-methyl-D-aspartate receptor antagonist MK-801. *Proc. Natl. Acad. Sci. USA* **89,** 5197–5200.

Oppenheimer R. W. (1991) Cell death during development of the nervous system. *Ann. Rev. Neurosci.* **14,** 453–501.

Poirier J. and Nichol N. R. (1991) Alteration of hippocampal RNA prevalence in response to deafferentation. *Methods Neurosci.* **7,** 182–199.

Poirier J., Baccichet A., Dea D., and Gauthier S. (1993) Cholesterol synthesis and lipoprotein uptake during synaptic remodelling in the hippocampus in adult rats. *Neuroscience* **55,** 81–90.

Poirier J., Hess M., May P. C., and Finch C. E. (1991) Apolipoprotein E and GFAP-RNA in hippocampus during reactive synaptogenesis and terminal proliferation. *Mol. Brain Res.* **11,** 97–106.

Randall R. D. and Thayer S. A. (1992) Glutamate–induced calcium transient triggers delayed calcium overload and neurotoxicity in rat hippocampal neurons. *J. Neurosci.* **12,** 1882–1895.

Sakhi S., Bruce A., Sun N., Tocco G., Baudry M., and Schreiber S. S. (1994) p53 induction is associated with neuronal damage in the central nervous system. *Proc. Natl. Acad. Sci. USA* **91,** 7525–7529.

Scheff S. W., Benardo L. S., and Cotman C. W. (1980) Decline in reactive fiber growth in the dentate gyrus of aged rats compared to young adult rats following entorhinal cortex removal. *Brain Res.* **199,** 21–38.

Schipper H. M. and Wang E. (1990) Expression of statin in the postnatal brain: evidence for a substantial retention of neuroglial proliferative capacity with aging. *Brain Res.* **528,** 250–258.

Schipper H. M., Skalski V., Panasci L. C., and Wang E. (1990) Statin expression in the untreated and SarCNU-exposed human glioma cell line, SK-MG-1. *Cancer Chemother. Pharmacol.* **26,** 383–386.

Schmidt-Kastner R. and Freund T. F. (1991) Selective vulnerability of the hippocampus in brain ischemia. *Neuroscience* **40,** 599–636.

Sester U., Sawada M., and Wang E. (1990) Purification and biochemical characterization of statin, a non-proliferation specific protein from rat liver. *J. Biol. Chem.* **265,** 19,966–19,972.

Shaw P., Bovey R., Tardy S., Sahli R., Sordat B., and Costa J. (1992) Induction of apoptosis by wild-type p53 in a human colon tumor-derived cell line. *Proc. Natl. Acad. Sci. USA* **89,** 4495–4499.

Sloviter R. S. and Lowenstein D. H. (1992) Heat shock protein expression in vulnerable cells of the rat hippocampus as an indicator of excitation–induced neuronal stress. *J. Neurosci.* **12,** 3004–3009.

Smith P. K., Krohn R. I., Hermanson G. T., Mallia A. K., Gartner F. H., Provenzano M. D., Fujimoto E. K., Goeke N. M., Olson B. J., and Klenk D. C. (1985) Measurement of protein using bicinchoninic acid. *Anal. Biochem.* **150,** 76–85.

Trump B. F. and Berezesky I. K. (1992) Role of cytosolic Ca^{2+} in cell injury necrosis and apoptosis. *Curr. Opinion Cell Biol.* **4,** 227–232.

Tsanaclis A. M. C., Brem S. S., Gately S., Schipper H. M., and Wang E. (1991) Statin immunolocalization in human brain tumors. *Cancer* **68,** 786–792.

Ulas J., Monaghan D. T., and Cotman C. W. (1990a) Plastic response of hippocampal excitatory amino acid receptors to deafferentation and reinnervation. *Neuroscience* **34,** 9–17.

Ulas J., Monaghan D. T., and Cotman C. W. (1990b) Kainate receptors in the rat hippocampus: a distribution and time course of changes in response to unilateral lesions of the entorhinal cortex. *J. Neurosci.* **10**, 2352–2362.

Van Hoesen G. W., Hyman B. T., and Damasio A. R. (1991) Entorhinal cortex pathology in Alzheimer's disease. *Hippocampus* **1**, 1–8.

Wang E. (1985) Rapid disappearance of statin, a nonproliferating and senescent cell-specific protein, upon reentering the process of cell cycling. *J. Cell Biol.* **101**, 1695–1701.

Wang E. (1989) Statin, a nonproliferation-specific protein, is associated with the nuclear envelope and is heterogenously distributed in cells leaving quiescent state. *J. Cell. Physiol.* **140**, 418–426.

Wang E. and Krueger J. G. (1985) Application of a unique monoclonal antibody as a marker for nonproliferating subpopulations of cells of some tissues. *J. Histochem. Cytochem.* **33**, 587–594.

Wang E. and Lin S. L. (1986) Disappearance of statin, a protein marker for nonproliferating and senescent cells following serum-stimulated cell cycle entry. *Exp. Cell Res.* **167**, 135–143.

Wang E., Lee M.-J., and Pandey S. (1994) Control of fibroblast senescence and activation of programmed cell death. *J. Cell. Biochem.* **54**, 432–439.

White W. F., Nadler J. V., Hamberger A., and Cotman C. W. (1977) Glutamate as transmitter of hippocampal perforant path. *Nature* **270**, 356,357.

Whitfield J. F. (1992) Calcium signals and cancer. *Curr. Rev. Oncol. Hematol.* **3**, 55–90.

Yonish–Rouach E., Resnitzky D., Lotem J., Sachs L., Kimchi A., and Oren M. (1991) Wild-type p53 induces apoptosis of myeloid leukaemic cells that is inhibited by interleukin-6. *Nature* **352**, 345–347.

Zhang X., Colombel M., Raffo A., and Buttyan R. (1994) Enhanced expression of p53 mRNA and protein in the regressing rat ventral prostate gland. *Biochem. Biophys. Res. Commun.* **198**, 1189–1194.

Zhang P., Hirsch E. C., Damier P., and Agig Y. (1992) C-fos protein-like immunoreactivity distribution in the human brain and over-expression in the hippocampus of patients with Alzheimer's disease. *Neuroscience* **49**, 9–21.

β-Amyloid-Induced Neuronal Cell Death in Transgenic Mice and Alzheimer's Disease

Frank M. LaFerla and Gilbert Jay

1. Introduction

Apoptosis plays a crucial role in tissue sculpturing during development and in the maintenance of a steady state in continuously renewing tissues. It is now becoming increasingly clear that apoptosis also contributes to cell death in many different pathological situations, including neurodegenerative disorders such as Alzheimer's disease (Su et al., 1994; Lassmann et al., 1995; LaFerla et al., 1995c) and infectious disorders like the acquired immunodeficiency syndrome (AIDS) (Meyaard et al., 1992; Gougeon and Montagnier, 1993). In this review, we will focus on the technical considerations that are critical for detecting apoptotic cells. Particular attention will be devoted to recently developed molecular techniques that offer enhanced detection of dying cells in tissue sections or in cell culture, especially as related to their utility in the brain.

Numerous review articles have detailed the morphological changes that occur in cells undergoing apoptosis (Majno and Joris, 1995) and, thus, these changes will only be described briefly here. Morphologically, apoptotic cells shrink and become denser, and the chromatin material becomes pyknotic and marginated against the nuclear membrane. This is accompanied by the internucleosomal degradation of cellular DNA, which

From: *Neuromethods, Vol. 29: Apoptosis Techniques and Protocols*
Ed: J. Poirier Humana Press Inc.

is considered the hallmark of the apoptotic process and yields a ladder-like DNA pattern when analyzed by gel electrophoresis (Arends et al., 1990). Eventually, the nucleus disintegrates (karyorhexis) and the cell emits processes that contain pyknotic nuclear fragments. It is generally thought that the cellular membrane remains intact throughout the entire process, enclosing organelles and contents of the dying cell, thereby reducing inflammation. An important feature of this, cell death process is the requirement for protein synthesis. Whereas these may be considered general characteristics of cells undergoing apoptosis, it is important to emphasize that the process may vary depending on the cell type. For instance, in many cells, DNA fragmentation appears to be a relatively early phenomenon, although in other cell types it clearly occurs much later in the process (Zakeri et al., 1993).

The ability to detect dying cells, particularly in tissue sections, affords the opportunity to investigate the pathogenic circumstances that lead to the demise of the cell. The identification of dying cells by morphological criteria alone is difficult, as processing artifacts introduced by different fixation regiments may affect the judgment. Several enzymatic methods have been employed to detect apoptosis at the single-cell level by capitalizing on the fragmented nature of the DNA to add labeled or conjugated nucleotides to either the 5' or 3' end. Essentially, these techniques involve either the tailing of the DNA by terminal deoxynucleotidyl transferase (TdT) (Gavrielli et al., 1992), referred to as the TUNEL method (TdT-biotin dUTP nick-end labeling), or nick-translation with DNA polymerase I or the Klenow fragment (Wijsman et al., 1993) or with T7 DNA polymerase (Wood et al., 1993), referred to as *in situ* end-labeling (ISEL) or *in situ* nick-translation (ISNT) (Gold et al, 1993). Both the TUNEL and ISEL methods have been extensively used by many investigators to detect apoptotic cells *in situ*.

These *in situ* labeling methods facilitate the study of apoptosis at the cellular level in tissue sections and cell culture systems, a comparison of the extent of involvement between affected areas, the detection of a single dying cell among a background of normal cells, and the identification of the precise cell type undergoing apoptosis or the factors that contributed to the cell death in combination with other marker analyses. Importantly, these molecular techniques identify dying cells at a level of sensitivity below the threshold for detecting DNA alterations-induced by autolysis or tissue processing artifacts (Lassmann et al., 1995).

In principle, these enzymatic techniques can detect all DNA breaks. Since the DNA is also fragmented in necrotic cells, these cells could conceptually be labeled by these biochemical procedures. In a recent comparison of the two techniques, the tailing method was found to be superior to nick-translation for the detection of apoptotic cells; in contrast, necrotic cells, in which the DNA is randomly fragmented, were preferentially labeled by nick-translation (Gold et al., 1994). Since the DNA in necrotic cells presumably accumulate more double-strand breaks than single strand breaks, the exonucleolytic activity of DNA polymerase I must be used to sufficiently amplify the signal at the site of the rare single-strand breaks; as a result, nick-translation is inferior to TUNEL in labeling apoptotic cells. The authors caution that since apoptotic cells are not at a synchronous stage in a given tissue and since the tailing method could label very late stage necrotic cells, they recommend the combined use of both techniques on serial sections to avoid any ambiguity. However, the TUNEL assay in combination with other morphologic or biochemical criteria, could allow the discrimination of apoptotic cells from necrotic cells.

2. The TUNEL Procedure

The tailing reaction is performed essentially as described by Gavrielli et al. (1992). Paraffin sections are dewaxed, rehydrated through a graded alcohol series, and digested with proteinase K (20 µg/mL). Endogenous peroxidase activity is quenched by treatment with hydrogen peroxide. Tissue sections are then rinsed and labeled at 37°C for 30–60 min with TdT in a cocktail consisting of 25 mM Tris, pH 6.6, 200 mM

potassium cacodylate, 1 mM cobalt chloride, 0.25 mg/mL bovine serum albumin, and 2 μM biotin-16-dUTP. The concentration of the TdT enzyme may vary depending on the tissue, although it is typically used in the range of 0.2–0.5 U/μL. After the enzymatic labeling, sections are rinsed and immersed in PBS and incubated with avidin and 3 biotinylated horseradish peroxidase for 15 min and then briefly rinsed and stained with diaminobenzidine (DAB, Vector Laboratories, Burlingame, CA) or True Blue (Kirkegaard & Perry, Gaithersburg, MD).

There are several factors that must be taken into consideration when attempting to label dying cells in tissues. Of paramount concern is the quality of the tissue samples. The postmortem period to fixation should be as short as possible to retain the integrity of the tissue and to reduce any artifactual DNA damage caused by autolysis. Additionally, the degree to which DNA breaks are accessible is partially dependent on protean digestion, which is tissue dependent; the optimal concentration and conditions must be carefully titrated for each tissue type. For mouse and human brain, we find that proteinase K digestion at 20 μg/mL for 20 min works well.

3. Alzheimer's Disease

Alzheimer's disease is a neurodegenerative disorder that is clinically characterized by progressive deterioration of memory and cognition. The prominent histopathological features of this disease include the intracellular accumulation of neurofibrillary tangles and the extracellular deposition of amyloid in specific regions of the brain; the principal constituent of the amyloid is a small peptide 39–43 amino acids in length, called β-amyloid or Aβ, which is derived from the amyloid precursor protein (APP) (Selkoe, 1995). The principal underlying cellular features of Alzheimer's disease are the degeneration and eventual death of neuronal cells in selective brain regions, such as the hippocampus, cerebral cortex, and amygdala; regions of the brain which play major roles in memory, behavior, and cognition. This cell loss, which accounts for many of the neurological deficits that are encountered, can be so profound, that at the time of death, the brain from an individual with Alzheimer's disease may weigh as little as one-half the weight of a normal, aged-matched control (Tomlinson, 1992).

Although the Aβ peptide has been the focus of much attention, its precise role in the pathophysiology of Alzheimer's disease remains unclear. The identification of missense mutations in *APP* and its association with early onset Alzheimer's disease certainly implicate the Aβ peptide in the disease process. To better understand the physiological role of Aβ in vivo, we used the neuronal-specific neurofilament-light *(NF-L)* promoter to drive expression of Aβ in transgenic mice. These NF_L-Aβ transgenic mice develop a subset of the pathological features that occur in Alzheimer's disease, including neuronal cell death, sparse extracellular amyloid deposition, reactive astrogliosis and microgliosis, seizures, and premature death (LaFerla et al., 1995a).

4. Aβ Expression Induces Apoptosis in Transgenic Mice

In the transgenic mice, the apoptotic death of neuronal cells occurs in selective regions of the brain, particularly in the hippocampus, cerebral cortex, thalamus, and amygdala. Not only do apoptotic cells occur in selective brain regions, but within a given region, selective areas consistently appear more vulnerable. This point is illustrated in the hippocampus and cerebral cortex shown in Fig. 1A,B, respectively. In this hippocampus from a transgenic mouse stained with TUNEL, the CA1 cells are profoundly affected, the CA3 cells are affected to a lesser degree, whereas cells of the CA2 tract and dentate gyrus are minimally involved. This situation is analogous in the cerebral cortex, where the superficial cortical layers are more affected compared to the deeper layers. In addition, a greater number of apoptotic cortical cells are present on the left side of this subregion. Moreover, apoptotic cells are intermingled with apparently healthy cells as

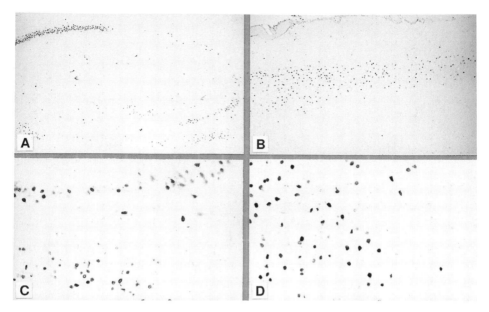

Fig. 1. Labeling of nuclei with fragmented DNA in Aβ-transgenic brains. The hippocampus **(A,C)** and cerebral cortex **(B,D)** from a 9-mo-old transgenic mouse stained with TUNEL. Original magnifications = 25×, A, B; 100×, C, D.

TUNEL-positive cells are juxtaposed to TUNEL-negative cells; this intermingling suggests that the TUNEL reaction is not labeling every cell in a nonspecific fashion and imparts a degree of confidence to the results.

The various stages of the apoptotic process can even be highlighted with the TUNEL reaction as shown in the high magnification photographs of the same two brain regions as above (Fig. 1C,D). Cells in which the nuclei are not yet condensed are visible, as are cells in which the chromatin has settled along the nuclear membrane, and even cells with highly condensed, pyknotic nuclei are quite readily apparent.

The demonstration that neuronal cells in the transgenic brains were undergoing apoptosis prompted us to ask whether a functional correlation could be established with the Aβ peptide. This type of analysis might indicate if cells needed to accumulate Aβ to die or whether downstream events might

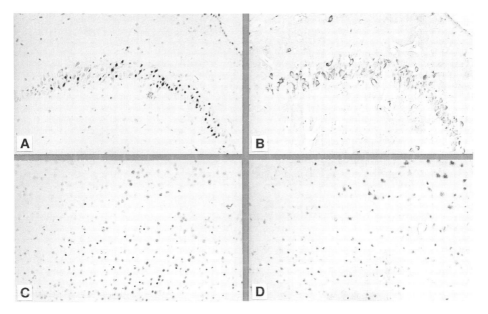

Fig. 2. *p53*-dependent neuronal cell death in Aβ-transgenic mice. Serial brain sections were stained with TUNEL **(A,C)** or with a *p53* antibody **(B,D)**. The hippocampus (A,B) and cerebral cortex (C,D) show that expression of p53 precedes cell death. Original magnification = 100×.

trigger nonexpressing cells to die. In fact, the former situation appears to be true as a good correlation can be established between neuronal cells undergoing apoptosis and the intracellular accumulation of Aβ, as shown in serial sections of the brain stained with TUNEL or anti-Aβ antibodies (Fig. 2A,B). Neuronal cells with prominent cytoplasmic Aβ staining have nuclei that are beginning to exhibit some TUNEL-reactivity; Aβ immunostaining appears much sparser in those cells with highly condensed nuclei (compare cells on the right tract to those on the left in Fig. 2A,B). This suggests that Aβ accumulation in these cells can induce programmed cell death. Although Aβ RNA expression occurs throughout the brain, accumulation of the Aβ peptide occurs in select neuronal cells. We hypothesize that some cellular cofactor may be required to stabilize the Aβ peptide intracellularly, allowing it to accumulate to levels sufficient to induce apoptosis.

Although we heavily relied on the TUNEL assay to initially characterize dying cells *in situ*, this was certainly not the only criterion we used. A combination of biochemical, morphological, and ultrastructural analyses were employed and provided a higher degree of confidence in determining if a cell was undergoing apoptosis. Our next goal was to define the underlying molecular mechanism that culminates in apoptosis of the Aβ containing neurons.

Over the past five years, many cellular genes have been shown to regulate apoptosis. Dissecting the molecular pathway by which apoptosis proceeds in response to a pathological stimulus (i.e., Aβ) in this animal model is not only of interest because of its relevance to Alzheimer's disease, but may even have broader implications for the field of apoptosis. Conceptually, apoptosis may proceed either through the activation of genes that promote cell death or through the inactivation of genes that suppress the death process, or through a combination of both. Many genes have been implicated in the apoptotic pathway (Korsmeyer, 1995), including *bc1-2, p53, bax, bcl-x, ICE, c-myc*, and *fas*, although not all have been shown to play a role in neurons. Some genes such as *bc1-2*, which are expressed in the brain in neonates and immature mice, do not appear to be expressed in the brain of adult animals to any significant level. Consequently, it is unlikely that *bc1-2* expression, which has been associated with promoting cell survival, will be altered in the brains of the transgenic mice.

One candidate gene we suspected might be involved in this transgenic system was *p53* (LaFerla et al., 1995b). The *p53* protein is a pleiotropic molecule that has been shown to be involved in programmed cell death, suppressing cell growth, and facilitating DNA repair (Oren, 1994). The involvement of *p53* has been demonstrated in neurons in response to ischemia and excitotoxicity (Li et al., 1994; Sakhi et al., 1994). Immunohistochemical staining of brain sections with antibodies to *p53* revealed that this molecule, which is typically not present in a substantial level in the brain of control animals, was expressed in those regions of the transgenic brain containing apoptotic cells (*see* Fig. 2C,D). Thus, Aβ is capable of inducing *p53* in this system which presumably underlies the apoptotic cell death. The process by which Aβ induces *p53* is unclear, although Aβ is suspected of causing oxidative damage (Behl et al., 1994; Hensley et al., 1994; Shearman et al., 1994) and *p53* is known to respond to this stimulus (Tishler et al., 1993).

5. Neurons Die by Apoptosis in Alzheimer's Disease Brains

The key observation that emerged from the study of this transgenic system was that intracellular Aβ expression was capable of promoting the apoptotic cell death of neurons. This finding prompted us to conduct an analysis of post-mortem brain tissues from Alzheimer's disease patients for concurrence. Characterizing the process by which neurons die in Alzheimer's disease is important as the clinical manifestations of-this disease stem from the dysfunction and death of neurons in selective regions of the brain.

Before we initiated these studies, we hypothesized that it might be difficult to demonstrate cell death in brain tissues from patients who died with advanced-stage disease, as the neuronal cells may have already been lost, and therefore would not label by TUNEL. In fact, in a patient with prominent neurohistological features of Alzheimer's disease, as defined by silver staining (Fig. 3B), many of the nuclei were no longer intact and those that were are only weakly labeled by TUNEL (Fig. 3A). In patients with less advanced neurohistological features (Fig. 3D), apoptosis of neurons as indicated by TUNEL are more readily apparent (Fig. 3C). In contrast, no TUNEL-positive cells were detected in the brains of control, nondemented individuals (Fig. 3E,F).

The apoptotic cells in the Alzheimer's disease brain exhibit distinct morphological changes. Accordingly, we were able to arbitrarily assign a particular stage to the cells based on the nuclear and cytoplasmic architecture. As shown in Fig. 4A, stage 1 cells were completely TUNEL-negative as they had no detectable DNA fragmentation within their

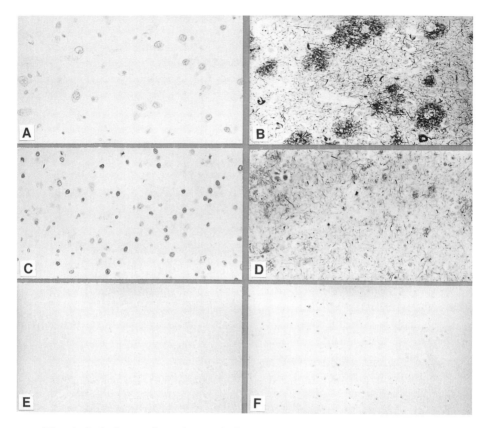

Fig. 3. Labeling of nuclei with fragmented DNA in Alzheimer's disease brains. The superior temporal gyrus from two AD patients (**A,B** and **C,D**, respectively) and from a control, nondemented individual (**E,F**), stained with either TUNEL (A,C,E) or Bielshowsky's silver stain (B,D,F) are shown. Original magnification = 100×.

nuclei and showed no discernable cytoplasmic region; these cells are essentially normal neurons. Stage 2 cells had slightly enlarged but normal appearing nuclei with variable amounts of TUNEL-staining due to the different extent of DNA fragmentation; this was accompanied by a marked expansion of the cytoplasmic compartment. We classify these cells as early-stage apoptotic cells. Stage 3 cells had TUNEL-positive nuclei that were somewhat condensed, in which the open chromatin morphology was no longer apparent and the cytoplasm

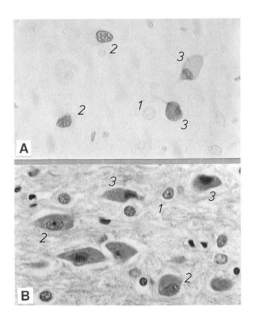

Fig. 4. Morphological changes in neurons of Alzheimer's disease brain sections as visualized by TUNEL **(A)** or hematoxylin-and-eosin staining **(B)**. The progression of nuclear and cytoplasmic changes are indicated by the numbers: stage 1 cells are essentially healthy appearing cells; stage 2 cells contain TUNEL-staining; stage 3 cells are TUNEL-positive with highly condensed nuclei and bacophilin cytoplasm. Original magnification = 200×.

appeared increasingly basophilic following hematoxylin-and-eosin staining. Stage 4 cells (not shown in this field) frequently had a crescent or panhandle shape where the collapsed TUNEL-positive nuclei appeared to be in the process of being extruded from one end of the cell; these are late-stage apoptotic cells. Occasionally, some of these later stage cells also show TUNEL-staining in the cytoplasm which we interpret to represent leakage of DNA fragments from the nucleus. This would then account for the basophilia that is observed in these cells.

In undertaking a postmortem analysis of tissue with TUNEL, we were cognizant of two factors that must be considered and that may affect the interpretation of our findings. First, postmortem changes in the Alzheimer's disease brain, including cell death, are sample specific and cannot simply be controlled by analysis of samples from uninvolved individuals. Second, the TUNEL method, although capable of detecting dying cells at different stages of the apoptotic pathway, cannot detect "dead" cells. To circumvent these concerns, we focused on regions that contained TUNEL-positive and TUNEL-negative cells juxtaposed to one another to ensure that the TUNEL reaction was not indiscriminately labeling cells. This precaution, in combination with the morphologic analysis, imparts a greater degree of confidence to our analysis.

References

Arends M. J., Morris R. G., and Wyllie A. H. (1990) Apoptosis. The role of the endonuclease. *Am. J. Pathol.* **136**, 593–608.

Behl C., Davis J. B., Lesley R., and Schubert D. (1994) Hydrogen peroxide mediates amyloid beta protein toxicity. *Cell* **77**, 817–827.

Butterfield D. A., Hensley K., Harris M., Mattson M., and Carney J. (1994) β-amyloid peptide free radical fragments initiate synaptosomal lipoperoxidation in a sequence-specific fashion: implications to Alzheimer's disease. *Biochem. Biophys. Res.* **200**, 710–715.

Gavrielli Y., Sherman Y., and Ben-Sasson S. A. (1992) Identification of programmed cell death *in situ* via specific labeling of nuclearDNA fragmentation. *J. Cell Biol.* **119**, 493–501.

Gold R., Schmied M., Giegerich G., Breitschopf H., Hartung H. P., Toyka K. V., and Lassmann H. (1994) Differentiation between cellular apoptosis and necrosis by the combined use of *in situ* tailing and nick translation techniques. *Lab. Invest.* **71**, 219–225.

Gold R., Schmied M., Rothe G., Zischler H., Breitschopf H., Wekerle H., and Lassmann H. (1993) Detection of DNA fragmentation in apoptosis: application of *in situ* nick translation to cell culture systems and tissue sections. *J. Histochem. Cytochem.* **41**, 1023–1030.

Gougeon M.-L. and Montagnier L. (1993) Apoptosis in AIDS. *Science* **260**, 1269,1270.

Haffner R. and Oren M. (1995) Biochemical properties and biological effects of p53. *Science* **5**, 84–90.

Hensley K., Carney J. M., Mattson M. P., Aksenova M., Harris M., Wu J. F., Floyd R. A., and Butterfien D. A. (1994) A model for β-amyloid aggregation and neurotoxicity based on free radical generation by the peptide: relevance to Alzheimer disease. *Proc. Natl. Acad. Sci. USA* **91**, 3270–3274.

Korsmeyer S. J. (1995) Regulators of cell death. *Trends Genet.* **11**, 101–105.

LaFerla F. M., Tinkle B. T., Bieberich C. J., Haudenschild C., and Jay G. (1995) The Alzheimer's Aβ peptide induces neurodegeneration and apoptosis in transgenic mice. *Nature Genetics* **9**, 21–30.

LaFerla F. M., Hall C. K., Ngo L., and Jany G. (1995b) Extracellular deposition of β-amyloid upon p53-dependent neuronal cell death in transgenic mice. Submitted.

LaFerla F. M., Troncoso J. C., Kawas C. H., and Jay G. (1995c) Apoptotic cell death precedes extracellular deposition of β-amyloid in Alzheimer's disease. *J. Clin. Invest.* **98**, 1626–1632.

Lassmann H., Bancher C., Breitschopf H., Wegiel J., Bobinski M., Jellinger K., and Wisniewski H. M. (1995) Cell death in Alzheimer's disease evaluated by DNA fragmentation *in situ*. *Acta Neuropathol.* **89**, 35–41.

Li Y., Chopp M., Zhang Z., Zaloga C., Niewenhuis L., and Gautam S. (1994) p53-immunoreactive protein and p53 mRNA expression after transient middle cereblral artery occlusion in rats. *Stroke* **25**, 849–856.

Majno G., and Joris I. (1995) Apoptosis oncosis, and necrosis: an overview of cell death. *Am. J. Pathol.* **146**, 3–15.

Meyaard L., Otto S. A., Jonker R. R., Mijinster M. J., Keet R. P. M., and Miedema F. (1992) Programmed death of T cells in HIV-1 infection. *Science* **257**, 217–219.

Sakhi S., Bruce A., Sun N., Tocco G., Baudry M., and Schreiber S. S. (1994) p53 induction is associated with neuronal damage in the central nervous system. *Proc. Natl. Acad. Sci. USA* **91**, 7525–7529.

Selkoe D. J. (1995) Deciphering Alzheimer's disease: molecular genetics and cell biology yield major clues. *J. NIH Res.* **7**, 57–64.

Shearman M. S., Ragan C. I., and Iversen L. L. (1994) Inhibition of PC 12 cell redox activity is a specific, early indicator of the mechanism of β-amyloid-mediated cell death. *Proc. Natl. Acad. Sci. USA* **91**, 1470–1474.

Tishler R. B., Calderwood S. K., Coleman C. N., and Price B. D. (1993) Increases in sequence specific DNA binding by p53 following treatment with chemotherapeutic and DNA damaging agents. *Cancer Res.* **53**, 2212–2216.

Tomlinson B. E. (1992) Ageing and the dementias in *Greenfield's Neuropathology*. Adams J. H. and Duchen L. W., eds., Oxford University Press, New York, pp. 1284–1410.

Wijsman J. H., Jonker R. R., Keijzer R., Van De Velde C. J. H., Cornelisse C. J., and Van Dierendonck J. H. (1993) A new method to detect apoptosis in paraffin sections: *in situ* end-labeling of fragmented DNA. *J. Histochem. Cytochem.* **411**, 7–12.

Wood K. A., Dipasquale B., and Youle R. J. (1993) *In situ* labeling of granule cells for apoptosis-associated DNA fragmentation reveals different mechanisms of cell loss in developing cerebellum. *Neuron* **11**, 621–632.

Zakeri Z. F., Quaglino D., Latham T., and Lockshin R. A. (1993) Delayed internucleosomal DNA fragmentation in programmed cell death. *FASEB J.* **7**, 470–478.

Use of TUNEL to Measure Retinal Ganglion Cell Apoptosis

Lisa Ayn Kerrigan and Donald J. Zack

1. Introduction

During development of the retina, a number of different cell types are produced in excess and then undergo programmed cell death (Young, 1984). Retinal ganglion cells, which are the tertiary neurons whose axons make up the optic nerve and provide connectivity between the eye and higher centers in the brain, are among those cells which die by programmed cell death (Rakic and Riley, 1983; Insausti et al., 1984; Provis and Penfold, 1988). The number of retinal ganglion cells that are born in the mammalian retina is approximately twice the number that survive. According to the neurotrophic hypothesis, the cells that die do so because they fail to receive the appropriate neurotrophic signal from their target tissue, in this case from the lateral geniculate nucleus (Cowan et al., 1984; Barde, 1989). This mechanism is thought to help ensure that inappropriate connections are not maintained and that the final steady-state number of innervating neurons is appropriately matched to the number of target cells.

Consistent with the neurotrophic hypothesis, retinal ganglion cells express neurotrophin receptors and respond to exogenous trophic factors. *In situ* hybridization and immunohistochemical experiments have shown that the receptor for the neurotrophin brain-derived neurotrophic factor (BDNF), trkB, is expressed by rat ganglion cells (Jelsma et al., 1993). In addition, BDNF has been reported to promote

From: *Neuromethods, Vol. 29: Apoptosis Techniques and Protocols*
Ed: J. Poirier Humana Press Inc.

ganglion cell survival both in vitro and in vivo (Johnson et al., 1986; Rodriguez et al., 1989; Mey and Thanos, 1993; Mansour-Robaey et al., 1994). Fibroblast growth factor, ciliary neurotrophic factor, and nerve growth factor also promote ganglion cell survival after injury (Sievers et al., 1987; Lipton et al., 1988; Lehwalder et al., 1989; Schulz et al., 1990; Siliprandi et al., 1993). Perhaps the most striking finding supportive of the applicability of the neurotrophic hypothesis to the death of retinal ganglion cells during development is the observation that transgenic mice that overproduce Bcl-2 have an approx 50% increase in ganglion cell number and a doubling of optic nerve surface area (Martinou et al., 1994).

Ganglion cell death due to loss of neurotrophic support does not occur only during development, but can also occur secondary to disease or trauma. Glaucoma, the third most prevalent cause of blindness worldwide (Thylefors and Negrel, 1994), is an optic neuropathy characterized by an excavated appearance of the optic nerve head and progressive loss of retinal ganglion cells (Quigley et al., 1981; Quigley et al., 1983; Quigley et al., 1991). Although the pathophysiology and underlying molecular mechanisms of glaucoma are not well understood, our hypothesis is that blockage of axoplasmic flow at the lamina cribrosa, which can be caused by increased intraocular pressure and has been observed in both human eyes with glaucoma and in experimental model systems (Anderson and Hendrickson, 1974; Quigley and Anderson, 1976; Minckler et al., 1977; Quigley et al., 1981), may cause a functional blockade of neurotrophic signaling from axonal terminals to ganglion cell bodies and thereby lead to cell death (Quigley et al., 1995). In an analogous manner, this same mechanism may account for the ganglion cell death observed after optic nerve transection.

As might be expected, since a variety of studies have implicated apoptosis as the mechanism of neuronal cell death associated with neurotrophin withdrawal (Batistatou and Green, 1991; Lindsay et al., 1994; Rubin et al., 1994), apoptosis has also been associated with retinal ganglion cell death during development (Portera-Cailliau et al., 1994), following optic nerve transection (Berkelaar et al., 1994; Garcia-Valenzuela et al., 1994; Quigley et al., 1995), and with animal models of glaucoma (Garcia-Valenzuela et al., 1995; Quigley et al., 1995). In our studies we have concentrated on morphological and TUNEL (terminal deoxynucleotidyl transferase (TdT)-mediated dUTP-biotin nick-end labeling) (Gavrieli et al., 1992) based evidence of apoptotic cell death (Fig. 1) (Quigley et al., 1995). In this chapter we will present a brief overview of the TUNEL method and then provide a detailed protocol of the modified method we use to study ganglion cell apoptosis in the retina.

2. The TUNEL Method: General Principle

Apoptosis is generally characterized by chromatin condensation, intracellular fragmentation associated with membrane-enclosed cellular fragments (apoptotic bodies), and internucleosomal DNA fragmentation (Kerr et al., 1972; Wyllie et al., 1984; Ellis et al., 1991). The presence of internucleosomal DNA fragmentation can usually be detected by the appearance of a "ladder" pattern on DNA gel electrophoresis (Wyllie, 1980), but this method does not allow the identification of individual cells undergoing apoptosis and, in some cases, the ladder pattern can be difficult to detect, especially if the proportion of cells undergoing apoptosis is very small. The TUNEL method was designed as a histochemical technique to detect internucleosomal DNA fragmentation at the level of individual cells (Gavrieli et al., 1992; Ben-Sasson et al., 1995). It relies on the *in situ* labeling of DNA breaks within nuclei. The method is based on the specific binding of TdT to the exposed 3'-OH ends of DNA fragments which are generated during the process of apoptosis. The TdT is a nontemplate-dependent DNA polymerase that catalyzes the addition of deoxyribonucleoside triphosphates to the 3' ends of double- or single-stranded DNA. To perform the TUNEL technique, histologic tissue sections or cell preparations are subjected to proteolytic treatment, followed by TdT to incorporate biotinylated deoxyuridine at the sites of DNA breaks. In order to enable histochemical visualization by light microscopy, the signal is amplified by avidin-peroxidase.

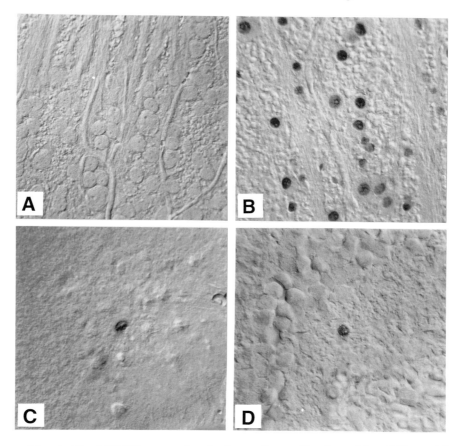

Fig. 1. The TUNEL-treated retinal ganglion cells viewed by differential interference contrast microscopy in sections cut parallel to the retinal surface. The appearance of normal retina is shown in **(A)**, with round ganglion cell nuclei, bundles of axons, and retinal capillaries. No TUNEL-positive cells are present. The positive control specimen **(B)** is a normal retina that was reacted with DNase I prior to the TUNEL reaction. The expected uniform red-brown positive reaction product is seen in the cell nuclei of the ganglion cell layer. **(C)** and **(D)** show TUNEL-positive cells present in a retina from a monkey with experimental glaucoma. (Quigley et al., 1995; reprinted with permission from Investigative Ophthalmology and Visual Science.)

2.1. Tissue Preparation

Fixation of the tissue can have dramatic effects on the cellular morphology of histologic sections. Ideally, tissue should be fixed with 4% buffered paraformaldehyde or formaldehyde for 1–7 d (Ben-Sasson et al., 1995); however, tissue which has been in fixative for extended periods of time, up to years, can also be used. Tissue fixation with 4% paraformaldehyde combined with 5% glutaraldehyde also works well (Quigley et al., 1995).

After fixation, tissue should be embedded in paraffin. Paraffin sections, generally 5–10 μm thick, should be cut in an orientation that maximizes the number of cells visible per slide. For retinal ganglion cells, sections can be cut parallel to the retinal surface to achieve the highest density of cells per slide (Quigley et al., 1995). The TUNEL method can also be applied to frozen sections; however, the proteolytic treatment should be decreased or omitted (Ben-Sasson et al., 1995).

When mounting paraffin sections on slides, it is important to use an appropriate adhesive to avoid loss of sections during the subsequent washing procedures. Sections can be mounted on Superfrost slides (Fisher Scientific, Pittsburgh, PA) or on glass slides that have been coated (subbed) with either 3-aminopropyl triethoxysilane (TESPA; No. A3648, Sigma, St. Louis, MO) or poly-L-lysine (300,000 mol wt; Sigma). TESPA has been shown to be superior to poly-L-lysine in preventing tissue detachment from the glass (Ben-Sasson et al., 1995). We have found Superfrost slides to be ideal since no subbing procedure is necessary and detachment of tissue is rare.

2.2. Proteolytic Treatment with Proteinase K

Tissue sections are partially deproteinized by incubation with Proteinase K. Proteinase K digests cross-linked proteins and thereby increases cell permeability and access to the nucleic acid targets (DNA). Proteinase K is preferred because it does not require predigestion to reduce residual nucleases (Wilson and Higgins, 1990). The concentration of proteinase K is extremely important. High concentrations can cause tissue damage and increase nonspecific staining (Tornusciolo et al., 1995).

Since the final immunohistochemical stain is peroxidase-based, endogenous peroxidases can produce high levels of background staining, which interfere with interpretation of results. To prevent this problem, endogenous peroxidases are inactivated by immersing slides in 3% H_2O_2.

2.3. Terminal Deoxynucleotidyl Transferase (TdT)

In the TUNEL method, TdT is used to incorporate biotinylated deoxyuridine at the sites of DNA breaks. Both single-stranded DNA and 3' overhangs of double-stranded DNA are good substrates for TdT. The TdT is generally inefficient at catalyzing the transfer of biotinylated dUTP to blunt or recessive ends (Deng and Wu, 1983). To increase sensitivity with blunt-ends and 5'-overhangs, the TUNEL method uses a cobalt-based buffer that allows higher efficiency tailing (Roychoudhury and Wu, 1980).

The TdT buffer is more effective if it is made fresh for each TUNEL reaction. To maximize efficiency, the TdT buffer can be made during the 15 min proteinase K incubation. The TdT buffer consists of cobalt chloride (Sigma), sodium cacodylate (Sigma), 30 mM Tris, pH 7.2, and sterile DDW. The TdT buffer is used for a preincubation step, for DNase controls, and for the terminal transferase/biotin labeling mixture. The amount of TdT buffer required for each slide depends on the amount of tissue adhered to the slide. For retinal sections of approx 10×10 mm, at least 40 μL per slide is required to prevent damage to the tissue. In order to ensure equal distribution of TdT buffer over the entire sample, a coverslip is applied to each slide. Damage can occur when coverslips are removed if an insufficient amount of buffer is used. Inadequate amounts of buffer can also cause the tissue to dry out. It is critical that the tissue does not dry out.

Before the preincubation step, the stock TdT buffer should be divided into aliquots necessary for the preincubation step, DNase controls and the TdT/biotin labeling mixture. For retinal sections, we aliquot 1 mL of TdT buffer for the DNase controls, and 400 mL for the labeling mixture. The remaining TdT buffer is used for the preincubation step. During preincubation, all experimental slides are covered with TdT buffer, coverslipped, and incubated in a humid chamber for 10 min at room temperature. While experimental slides are being covered with TdT and coverslipped, designated DNase control slides should remain in DDW in order to prevent tissue damage. Positive DNase control slides should be processed immediately after the experimental slides are placed in the humid chamber. Experimental slides should not be removed from the humid chamber until after DNase control slides have been processed and thoroughly washed with DDW.

2.4. Positive DNase Controls

There is a substantial amount of variation in positive staining when using the TUNEL method; therefore, at least two DNase control slides should be included with each experimental run (Fig. 1B). The type, size, and fixation of the tissue are contributing factors to the variation in staining. Since DNA fragmentation is characteristic of apoptosis, application of DNase I to control slides is ideal. DNase I is an endonuclease that introduces breaks by hydrolyzing double-stranded, or single-stranded DNA, preferentially at sites adjacent to pyrimidine nucleotides (Sambrook et al., 1989); therefore, pretreatment with DNase I results in intensive labeling of all nuclei. If the DNase I controls do not stain, staining on the experimental slides may be artifact and not positive staining.

To make the DNase I mixture, 4 µL of RNase-free DNase I (Boehringer Mannheim, Mannheim, Germany) is added to 1 mL of TdT buffer. After finger flicking for 10 s, the DNase mixture should be applied to the desired DNase control slides. This mixture should not be made until needed since thawing of the DNase I causes its inactivation. After DNase I pretreatment, all slides should be washed thoroughly with DDW, since residual DNase activity can introduce high background.

2.5. TdT/Biotin Reaction Mixture

Elongation of the DNA fragments occurs during incubation in the TdT/biotin reaction mixture. The TdT/biotin labeling mixture should not be made until after DNase controls have been rinsed with DDW. The labeling mixture consists of 2 μL TdT (Boehringer Manheim) and 4 μL biotin 16-dUTP (Boehringer Manheim) per 100 μL TdT buffer (made fresh). Biotin-11–dUTP or digoxygenin-conjugates of dNTP can be used instead of biotin-16-dUTP (Ben-Sasson et al., 1995). Coverslips and excess fluid should be removed from experimental slides and the labeling mixture should be applied to both experimental and DNase slides simultaneously. All slides should incubate coverslipped for 60 min at 37°C in a humid chamber. Both experimental and DNase control slides should be processed together for the remaining steps.

2.6. Termination of Reaction

The reaction is terminated by immersing the slides in 2X SSC (300 m*M* NaCl and 30 m*M* sodium citrate, pH 8.0) for 15 min at room temperature. Next, the slides are washed in phosphate-buffered saline (PBS) for 15 min at room temperature. Blocking is accomplished by covering sections with 2% bovine serum albumin (BSA) in PBS for 10 min at room temperature. Human serum albumin has also been successfully used as a blocking agent (Ben-Sasson et al., 1995). Excess albumin is removed by incubating the slides in PBS for 5 min at room temperature.

2.7. ABC Staining

We prefer the avidin-conjugated peroxidase-based Vectastain ABC Kit (Vector Laboratories, Burlingame, CA) for staining with the TUNEL method. The kit contains Avidin DH and biotinylated horseradish peroxidase H reagents that form a complex that is ideal for immunoperoxidase staining. Even though the structure of the complex is not well defined, it is thought to consist of many biotinylated horseradish peroxidase molecules crosslinked by avidin. Avidin is a glycoprotein with an extremely high affinity for biotin. The affinity is so high that the binding of avidin to biotin is essentially irreversible. The ABC technique consists of an unlabeled primary antibody, a biotinylated secondary antibody followed by an avidin and biotinylated horseradish peroxidase complex.

The ABC reagent should be made 30 min prior to use. The ABC reagent consists of 50 µL of solution A, 50 µL of solution B, and 5 µL of PBS. Sections should be incubated in the ABC reagent (100 µL per slide) and coverslipped for 30 min in a humid chamber at 37°C.

Fluorescent-labeled (FITC) avidin can be used instead of peroxidase-avidin for fluorescence microscopy, but it does not have the advantage of enzymatic amplification (Ben-Sasson et al., 1995).

2.8. AEC Staining

There are several chromogens that can act as electron donors for immunoperoxidase techniques. The 3-amino-9-ethylcarbazole (AEC) is one of the most commonly used chromogens. The AEC forms a red endproduct that is alcohol soluble; therefore, sections should not be dehydrated. Sections should be coverslipped with a water-based medium such as Polymount (Polysciences, Warrington, PA). Glycerol-gelatin (Sigma) may also be used as a mounting media (Ben-Sasson et al., 1995). The coverslipped slides can be stored for many months at room temperature. The AEC is stable for 2–3 h after preparation. When AEC is dissolved in DMSO, the mixture is stable for long periods of time and can be stored as a stock solution for 2–3 mo. The AEC is light-sensitive; therefore, it should be stored in a dark environment. Care should be taken to avoid inhalation of the powder or contact with the skin because AEC may be a carcinogen.

3,3-Diaminobenzidine (DAB) and a nonaqueous mounting medium such as alkylacrylate in xylene may also be used for the TUNEL method (Ben-Sasson et al., 1995). One of the major drawbacks to using DAB is that it is a carcinogen. Another difference between AEC and DAB is the pH at which they are used. The AEC is used at pH 5.2, whereas DAB is used at pH 7.2. The lower pH may limit the amount of background staining in the tissue sections. Another way to limit the amount of background is to use strepavidin-peroxidase and extra-avidin peroxidase (BioMakor, Rehovot, Israel) rather than native egg avidin. Conjugated alkaline phosphatase along with the appropriate chromogen have also worked well (Ben-Sasson et al., 1995).

Slides should be stained in AEC substrate for at least 30 min at room temperature and then washed three times for 5 min each. After 30 min, the DNase controls should be checked for staining. If they are not stained, we suggest that the slides remain in the substrate for up to 90 min. Staining at 37°C for 30 min and washing with PBS can also be used (Ben-Sasson et al., 1995).

3. The TUNEL Method: Step-by-Step Procedure

3.1. Helpful Hints

1. During treatments, slides should be held in glass slide racks and immersed in glass staining dishes containing 250 mL of the indicated solutions unless otherwise specified.
2. All solutions should be made with sterile DDW.
3. Fresh solvents are recommended since paraffin residues may interfere with the enzymatic reaction.

3.2. Slides

If Superfrost slides are not used, slides should be subbed (with TESPA or poly-L-lysine) at least 2 d prior to application of paraffin sections. Two procedures for subbing slides are as follows:

3.2.1. TESPA

1. Dip slides in 10% HCl (FIX)/70% ethanol.
2. Dip slides in distilled water.
3. Dip slides in 95% ethanol.
4. Dry slides in an oven at 150°C for 15 min and allow to cool.
5. Dip slides in 2% TESPA in acetone for 10 s.
6. Wash twice with acetone.
7. Dip slides in distilled water.
8. Dry at 42°C.

3.2.2. Poly-L-Lysine

1. Acid clean slides overnight with 1.2*N* HCl in glass staining dish.
2. Rinse in running tap water for 1 h.
3. Rinse in running distilled water for 1 h.
4. Dip slides in poly-L-lysine/buffer for 10 min (50 mg poly-L-lysine in 500 mL 10 m*M* Tris, pH 8.0.).
5. Blot on bottom and air dry protected from dust.

3.2.3. Deparaffinizing Sections

Cut paraffin sections by standard methods. Paraffin slides can be stored at room temperature until use. Deparaffinizing the slides can be achieved by heating the slides for 1 h at 60°C (Quigley et al., 1995), for 10 min at 70°C, or for 30 min at 60°C (Gavrieli et al., 1992). Hydration of the tissue is accomplished by transferring the slides through the following washes:

1. Xylene (twice for 5 min each).
2. 100% ETOH (twice for 3 min each).
3. 95% ETOH (twice for 3 min each).
4. 90% ETOH for 3 min.
5. 80% ETOH for 3 min.
6. Distilled water (twice for 3 min each)

3.2.4. Deproteinization with Proteinase K

1. Immerse slides in 10 m*M* Tris-HCl, pH 8.0, for 5 min at room temperature.
2. Incubate in 20 µg/mL proteinase K/Tris (Sigma) for 15 min at room temperature (RT).
3. Wash in DDW four times for 2 min each.
4. Immerse in 3% H_2O_2 for 5 min at RT.
5. Rinse in DDW three times for 2 min each.

3.2.5. Terminal Transferase Labeling

1. The TdT buffer required for each experiment is as follows:
   a. 0.24 g cobalt chloride.
   b. 0.30g sodium cacodylate.

    c. 300 µL of stock 30 m*M* Tris, pH 7.2.

    d. QS to 10 mL with sterile DDW.

2. Place 40 µL TdT buffer on each experimental slide and coverslip.

3. Incubate at RT for 10 min in humid chamber (stay in humid chamber until washes for DNase controls are completed).

4. For DNase I controls add 4 µL of DNase I/RNase free (Boehringer Manheim) to 1 mL TdT buffer.

5. Apply 75 µL of DNase mixture to each positive control slide, coverslip, and incubate for 10 min in a humid chamber. (Do not let DNase I thaw.)

6. Rinse with DDW (twice for 2 min each).

7. Remove coverslips and excess fluid from all slides (experimental and control).

8. Add 40 µL TdT/biotin labeling mixture to each slide, coverslip, and incubate in a humid chamber at 37°C for 60 min. The labeling mixture consists of the following:

    a. 2 µL Terminal Transferase (Boehringer Manheim).

    b. 4 µL Biotin-16-dUTP (Boehringer Manheim).

    c. 100 µL TdT buffer (made fresh).

    Hints: Be sure to make enough labeling mixture to adequately cover tissue sections. For retinal sections, 40 µL of labeling mixture should be used for each slide. Do not make the labeling mixture until it is needed.

3.2.6. Termination of Reaction and Staining

1. Make ABC mixture immediately before terminating reaction. Use VectaStain ABC Kit. Add 50 µL A and 50 µL B from kit to 5 mL PBS.

2. Stop reaction with 2X SSC for 15 min at RT.

3. Wash for 15 min in PBS.

4. Block with 2% BSA in PBS for 10 min at RT.

5. Wash for 5 min in PBS.

6. Apply avidin-conjugated peroxidase (ABC mixture), coverslip and incubate at 37°C for 30 min in humid chamber (100 µL for each slide).
7. Stain with substrate for 30 min in a glass staining dish. Substrate:
    a. 24 mL AEC (3-amino-9-ethylcarbazole).
    b. 200 mL 0.25M NaAc pH 5.2.
    c. 1600 µL 30% H_2O_2.
8. Wash with DDW (three times for 5 min each).
9. Allow sections to air dry.
10. Coverslip with Polymount (PolySciences, Warrington, PA).

4. Related Methods

Recently, a number of modifications of the TUNEL method have been developed to expand its usefulness. Microwave irradiation of paraffin sections has been reported to increase the sensitivity of the assay (Strater et al., 1995). The TUNEL method has been combined with cell surface labeling using flow cytometry (Sgonc et al., 1994). The TUNEL method can also be performed in conjunction with immunohistochemical staining for assay of multiple markers in the same tissue section. Tornuscilio et al. have described the use of an immunogold-silver intensification TUNEL stain in combination with fluorescent antibodies to detect apoptosis, growth-associated protein-43 expression, and bromodeoxyuridine incorporation (Tornusciolo et al., 1995). Using this method, they reported the ability to simultaneously identify proliferative, differentiated, and apoptotic cells in the embryonic mouse nervous system.

Several companies now make kits for the performance of TUNEL and related assays. The authors do not have any experience or affiliation with the kits. Among the kits that we have recently seen advertisements for are: DNA Fragmentation Detection Kit (Calbiochem, La Jolla, CA), Apoptosis/DNA Fragmentation Detection Kit (Kamiya Biomedical Company, Thousand Oaks, CA), Apotag (Oncor, Gaithersburg, MD), and TACS Blue Label (Trevigen, Gaithersburg, MD).

As a word of caution, it should be remembered that TUNEL-based assays measure the availability of free DNA 3'-OH ends; they do not directly measure the presence of internucleosomal DNA fragmentation, which itself may not be exclusively limited to cells undergoing apoptosis. Thus, these methods should not be considered totally specific for apoptosis. In fact, in at least some cases, necrotic and autolytic cells have been reported to be TUNEL-positive (Grasl et al., 1995).

5. Summary and Conclusions

Despite the caveat just mentioned, TUNEL has proven to be a powerful method for the study of apoptosis at the single-cell level. Using TUNEL, apoptosis has been identified as a mechanism of retinal ganglion cell death following axotomy and in animal models of glaucoma (Berkelaar et al., 1994; Garcia-Valenzuela et al., 1994, 1995; Quigley et al., 1995). We are also pursuing similar studies of apoptosis in human glaucoma. TUNEL has also implicated apoptosis in the death of retinal photoreceptors during development, following retinal detachment, and in murine and transgenic models of retinal degeneration (Shahinfar et al., 1991; Huang et al., 1993; Adler et al., 1994; Portera-Cailliau et al., 1994; Chang et al., 1995).

Understanding the role of apoptosis in retinal development and disease will likely have clinical as well as scientific implications. Definition of apoptosis as the final common pathway of ganglion cell and photoreceptor cell death in glaucoma and retinal degenerations, respectively, could lead to the development of therapeutic approaches that block cell death by interfering with the apoptotic pathway. As noted in Section 1., transgenic mice that overexpress Bcl-2 demonstrate reduced ganglion cell programmed cell death (Martinou et al., 1994). Transgenic mice that overexpress Bcl-2 in their photoreceptors have been reported to exhibit reduced photoreceptor cell loss in a murine retinal degeneration model (Flannery et al., 1995). In addition, intraocular administration of neurotrophins has also been reported to reduce both ganglion cell and photoreceptor cell apoptosis (LaVail et al., 1992; Mey and Thanos, 1993; Steinberg, 1994; Unoki and LaVail, 1994). Through pharmacologic or gene therapy approaches, it may one day be possible to develop a common strategy for the treatment of a variety of retinal and optic nerve diseases (Zack, 1993; Adler, 1996).

Acknowledgments

The authors wish to thank Harry A. Quigley and Mary Ellen Pease for assistance in the preparation of this manuscript. This work was supported by grants from the National Institutes of Health, Glaucoma Foundation, American Health Assistance Foundation, and unrestricted funds from Research to Prevent Blindness and the Rebecca P. Moon, Charles M. Moon, Jr., and Dr. Thomas Manchester Research Fund.

References

Adler A., Chang C., Fu J., and Tso M. (1994) Photic injury triggers apoptosis of photoreceptor cells. *Invest. Ophthalmol. Vis. Sci.* **35**, 1517.

Adler R. (1996) Mechanisms of photoreceptor death in retinal degenerations. *Arch. Ophthalmol.* **111**, 79–83.

Anderson D. R. and Hendrickson A. (1974) Effect of intraocular pressure on rapid axoplasmic transport in monkey optic nerve. *Invest. Ophthalmol.* **13**, 771–783.

Barde Y. A. (1989) Trophic factors and neuronal survival. *Neuron* **2**, 1525–1534.

Batistatou A. and Green L. A. (1991) Internucleosomal DNA cleavage and neuronal survival/death. *J. Cell Biol.* **122**, 523–532.

Ben-Sasson S., Sherman Y., and Gavrieli Y. (1995) Indentification of dying cells—*in situ* staining, in *Methods in Cell Biology.* Schwartz L. and Osborne, B., eds., Academic, San Diego, pp. 29–39.

Berkelaar M., Clarke D. B., Wang Y. C., Bray G. M., and Aguayo A. J. (1994) Axotomy results in delayed death and apoptosis of retinal ganglion cells in adult rats. *J. Neurosci.* **14**, 4368–4374.

Chang C. J., Lai W. W., Edward D. P., and Tso M. O. (1995) Apoptotic photoreceptor cell death after traumatic retinal detachment in humans. *Arch. Ophthalmol.* **113**, 880–886.

Cowan W. M., Fawcett J. W., O'Leary D. D., and Stanfield B. B. (1984) Regressive events in neurogenesis. *Science* **225**, 1258–1265.

Deng G.-R. and Wu R. (1983) Terminal transferase: use in the tailing of DNA and for in vitro mutagenesis. *Methods Enzymol.* **100,** 96–116.

Ellis R. E., Yuan J. Y., and Horvitz H. R. (1991) Mechanisms and functions of cell death. *Ann. Rev. Cell Biol.* **7,** 663–698.

Flannery J., Chen J., Xu J., and Simon M. (1995) Overexpression of Bcl-2 can interfer with apoptosis in retinal degeneration. *Invest. Vis. Sci. Ophthalmol.* **36,** 2848.

Garcia-Valenzuela E., Gorczyca W., Darzynkiewicz Z., and Sharma S. (1994) Apoptosis in adult retinal ganglion cells after axotomy. *J. Neurobiol.* **25,** 431–438.

Garcia-Valenzuela E., Shareef S., Walsh J., and Sharma S. C. (1995) Programmed cell death of retinal ganglion cells during experimental glaucoma. *Exp. Eye Res.* **61,** 33–44.

Gavrieli Y., Sherman Y., and Ben S. S. (1992) Identification of programmed cell death *in situ* via specific labeling of nuclear DNA fragmentation. *J. Cell Biol.* **119,** 493–501.

Grasl K. B., Ruttkay N. B., Koudelka H., Bukowska K., Bursch W., and Schulte H. R. (1995) *In situ* detection of fragmented DNA (TUNEL assay) fails to discriminate among apoptosis, necrosis, and autolytic cell death: a cautionary note. *Hepatology* **21,** 1465–1468.

Huang P., Gaitan A., Hao Y., Petters R., and Wong F. (1993) Cellular interactions implicated in the mechanism of photoreceptor degeneration in transgenic mice expressing a mutant rhodopsin gene. *Proc. Natl. Acad. Sci. USA* **90,** 8484–8488.

Insausti R., Blakemore C., and Cowan W. M. (1984) Ganglion cell death during development of ipsilateratal retinocollicullar projection in golden hamster. *Nature* **308,** 362–365.

Jelsma T. N., Friedman H. H., Berkelaar M., Bray G. M., and Aguayo A. J. (1993) Different forms of the neurotrophin receptor trkB mRNA predominate in rat retina and optic nerve. *J. Neurobiol.* **24,** 1207–1214.

Johnson J. E., Barde Y. A., Schwab M., and Thoenen H. (1986) Brain–derived neurotrophic factor supports the survival of cultured rat retinal ganglion cells. *J. Neurosci.* **6,** 3031–3038.

Kerr J. F. K., Wyllie A. H., and Currie A. H. (1972) Apoptosis, a basic biological phenomenon with wider implications in tissue kinetics. *Br. J. Cancer* **26,** 239–245.

LaVail M. M., Unoki K., Yasumura D., Matthes M. T., Yancopoulos G. D., and Steinberg R. H. (1992) Multiple growth factors, cytokines, and neurotrophins rescue photoreceptors from the damaging effects of constant light. *Proc. Natl. Acad. Sci. USA* **89,** 11,249–11,253.

Lehwalder D., Jeffrey P. L., and Unsicker K. (1989) Survival of purified embryonic chick retinal ganglion cells in the presence of neurotrophic factors. *J. Neurosci. Res.* **24,** 329–337.

Lindsay R. M., Wiegand S. J., Altar C. A., and DiStefano P. S. (1994) Neurotrophic factors: from molecule to man. *Trends Neurosci.* **17,** 182–190.

Lipton S. A., Wagner J. A., Madison R. D., and D'Amore P. A. (1988) Acidic fibroblast growth factor enhances regeneration of processes by postnatal mammalian retinal ganglion cells in culture. *Proc. Natl. Acad. Sci. USA* **85,** 2388–2392.

Mansour-Robaey S., Clarke D. B., Wang Y. C., Bray G. M., and Aguayo A. J. (1994) Effects of ocular injury and administration of brain-derived neurotrophic factor on survival and regrowth of axotomized retinal ganglion cells. *Proc. Natl. Acad. Sci. USA* **91,** 1632–1636.

Martinou J., Duboisdauphin M., and Staple K. (1994) Overexpression of bcl-2 in transgenic mice protects neurons from naturally occuring cell death and experimental ischemia. *Neuron* **13,** 1017–1030.

Mey J. and Thanos S. (1993) Intravitreal injections of neurotrophic factors support the survival of axotomized retinal ganglion cells in adult rats in vivo. *Brain Res.* **602,** 304–317.

Minckler D. S., Bunt A. H., and Johanson G. W. (1977) Orthograde and retrograde axoplasmic transport during acute ocular hypertension in the monkey. *Invest. Ophthalmol. Vis. Sci.* **16,** 426–441.

Portera-Cailliau C., Sung C. H., Nathans J., and Adler R. (1994) Apoptotic photoreceptor cell death in mouse models of retinitis pigmentosa. *Proc. Natl. Acad. Sci. USA* **91,** 974–978.

Provis J. M. and Penfold P. L. (1988) Cell death and the elimination of retinal axons during development. *Prog. Neurobiol.* **31,** 331–347.

Quigley H., Brown A., and Dorman-Pease M. (1991) Alterations in elastin of the optic nerve head in human and experimental glaucoma. *Br. J. Ophthalmol.* **75,** 552–557.

Quigley H., Hohman R., Addicks E., and Green W. (1983) Morphologic changes in the lamina cribrosa correlated with neural loss in open-angle glaucoma. *Am. J. Ophthalmol.* **95,** 673–691.

Quigley H. A., Addicks E. M., Green W. R., and Maumenee A. E. (1981) Optic nerve damage in human glaucoma: II: the site of injury and susceptibility to damage. *Arch. Ophthalmol.* **99,** 635–649.

Quigley H. A. and Anderson D. R. (1976) The dynamics and location of axonal transport blockade by acute intraocular pressure elevation in primate optic nerve. *Invest. Ophthalmol.* **15,** 606–616.

Quigley H. A., Nickells R. W., Kerrigan L. A., Pease M. E., Thibault D. J., and Zack D. J. (1995) Retinal ganglion cell death in experimental glaucoma and after axotomy occurs by apoptosis. *Invest. Ophthalmol. Vis. Sci.* **36,** 774–786.

Rakic P. and Riley K. P. (1983) Overproduction and elimination of retinal axons in the fetal rhesus monkey. *Science* **219,** 1441–1444.

Rodriguez T. A., Jeffrey P. L., Thoenen H., and Barde Y. A. (1989) The survival of chick retinal ganglion cells in response to brain-derived neurotrophic factor depends on their embryonic age. *Dev. Biol.* **136,**

Roychoudhury R. and Wu R. (1980) Labeling of duplex DNA with terminal transferase. *Methods Enzymol.* **65,** 42–62.

Rubin L. L., Gatchalian C. L., Rimon G., and Brooks S. F. (1994) The molecular mechanisms of neuronal apoptosis. *Curr. Opinion Neurobiol.* **4,** 696–702.

Sambrook J., Fritsch E., and Maniatis T. (1989) *Molecular Cloning: A Laboratory Manual.* Cold Spring Laboratory Press, Cold Spring Harbor, NY.

Schulz M., Raju T., Ralston G., and Bennett M. R. (1990) A retinal ganglion cell neurotrophic factor purified from the superior colliculus. *J. Neurochem.* **55,** 832–841.

Sgonc R., Boeck G., Dietrich H., Gruber H., Recheis H., and Wick G. (1994) Simultaneous determination of cell surface antigens and apoptosis. *Trends Genet.* **10,** 41,42.

Shahinfar S., Edward D., and Tso M. (1991) A pathologic study of photoreceptor cell death in retinal photic injury. *Curr. Eye Res.* **10,** 47–59.

Sievers J., Hausmann B., Unsicker K., and Berry M. (1987) Fibroblast growth factors promote the survival of adult rat retinal ganglion cells after transection of the optic nerve. *Neurosci. Lett.* **76,** 157–162.

Siliprandi R., Canella R., and Carmignoto G. (1993) Nerve growth factor promotes functional recovery of retinal ganglion cells after ischemia. *Invest. Ophthalmol. Vis. Sci.* **34,** 3232–3245.

Steinberg R. H. (1994) Survival factors in retinal degenerations. *Curr. Opinion Neurobiol.* **4,** 515–524.

Strater J., Gunthert A. R., Bruderlein S., and Moller P. (1995) Microwave irradiation of paraffin-embedded tissue sensitizes the TUNEL method for *in situ* detection of apoptotic cells. *Histochem. Cell Biol.* **103,** 157–160.

Thylefors B. and Negrel A. (1994) The global impact of glaucoma. *Bull. World Health Organization* **72,** 323–326.

Tornusciolo D. R. Z., Schmidt R. E., and Roth K. A. (1995) Simultaneous detection of TdT-mediated dUTP-biotin nick-end-labeling (TUNEL)-positive cells and multiple immunohistochemical markers in single tissue sections. *BioTechniques* **19,** 800–805.

Unoki K. and LaVail M. M. (1994) Protection of the rat retina from ischemic injury by brain-derived neurotrophic factor, ciliary neurotrophic factor, and basic fibroblast growth factor. *Invest. Ophthalmol. Vis. Sci.* **35,** 907–915.

Wilson M. and Higgins G. (1990) *In situ* hybridization, in *Neuromethods.* Boulton A., Baker G., and Campagnoni A., eds., Humana, Clifton, NJ, pp. 239–284.

Wyllie A. (1980) Glucocorticoid-induced thymocyte apoptosis is associated with endogenous endonuclease activation. *Nature* **284,** 555.

Wyllie A. H., Morris R. G., Smith A. L., and Dunlop D. (1984) Chromatin cleavage in apoptosis: association with condensed cleavage in apoptosis: association with condensed chromatin morphologyand dependence on macromolecular synthesis. *J. Pathol.* **142,** 67–77.

Young R. W. (1984) Cell death during differentiation of the retina in the mouse. *J. Comp. Neurol.* **229,** 362–373.

Zack D. J. (1993) Ocular gene therapy. From fantasy to foreseeable reality. *Arch. Ophthalmol.* **111,** 1477–1479.

Methods for Detection
of Apoptosis in the CNS

Kathrin D. Geiger, Floyd E. Bloom, and Nora E. Sarvetnick

1. Introduction

Despite recent scientific advances, the mechanisms inducing neuronal death in many human brain diseases remain unknown. Selective neuronal vulnerability, often with slowly developing loss of neurons, is a common feature of neurodegenerative disorders, infectious CNS diseases and their postinfectious states, certain forms of epilepsy, and hypoxic injuries. The assessment of damage in the CNS is complicated by the finding that neurons, although selectively damaged, are not the only group of cells involved in disease processes within the brain. Neuronal death even may be a secondary event induced by loss of function in glial populations or secretion of neurotoxic substances such as cytokines. However, recent data suggest that one common mechanism of neuronal loss in several CNS diseases may be apoptosis, also known as programmed cell death.

2. Characteristics of Apoptosis

By definition, the term apoptosis relates to the morphological description of a process of delayed cell death in which the dying cell actively participates (Kerr et al., 1972) as opposed to necrosis—a pathologic event acting directly on the cell. Compared to necrosis, apoptosis is selective and char-

From: *Neuromethods, Vol. 29: Apoptosis Techniques and Protocols*
Ed: J. Poirier Humana Press Inc.

acterized by distinctive biochemical and morphological features, including chromatin condensation with nuclear pyknosis, internucleosomal DNA fragmentation, and cytoplasmic shrinkage (Kerr et al., 1987) while cellular membranes are still intact. The process of apoptosis is linked to regulation of the cell cycle, originating from the G0 phase (Ellis et al., 1991) and requires protein synthesis (Wyllie, 1980). Accordingly, inhibitors of macromolecular protein synthesis reduce the amount of delayed neuronal death after ischemic injury (Schreiber and Baudry, 1995).

3. Apoptosis in the CNS

Under normal circumstances, apoptosis has an important role in the developing brain, that of removing excess neurons (Ellis et al., 1991) or neurons not needed for differentiation (Oppenheimer et al., 1995). Outside the brain, apoptosis is known to occur in response to hormonal depletion (Kerr et al., 1987; Edwards et al., 1991; Pittman et al., 1994; Schreiber and Maudry, 1995) or toxic stimuli (Anderton et al., 1995; Schreiber and Maudry, 1995) and in some tumors (Freeman et al., 1993; Kronbluth, 1994; Ellison et al., 1995). Under pathological conditions, apoptosis has been demonstrated in multiple CNS diseases such as neurodegenerative diseases like morbus Alzheimer (Lassmann et al., 1995) and amyotrophic lateral sclerosis (Yoshiyama et al., 1994), infectious diseases like Prion disease (Giese and Hess, 1995; Jeffrey et al., 1995), and several viral infections (Müller et al., 1992; Griffin et al., 1994; Ubol et al., 1994; Geiger et al., 1995). Apoptosis of neurons can also be induced by interruption of normal biochemical pathways (Ellis et al., 1987; Schreiber and Baudry, 1995) and by a range of "toxic" substances, including antimetabolites used in cytostatic therapy (Schreiber and Baudry, 1995), heat-shock proteins (Schreiber and Baudry, 1995), kainate (Ferrer et al., 1995), and several cytokines (Mangan et al., 1992; Fluckiger et al., 1994; Geiger et al., 1995). The sulfated glycoprotein clusterin is probably also involved in the generation of apoptosis (Schreiber and Baudry, 1995). Additionally, neurotransmitter analogs used for experimental generation of morbus Parkinson, such as 6-hydroxydopamine and MPP^+ (Mochizuki et al., 1994; Walkinshaw and Water, 1994), are known to induce apoptosis.

4. Possible Mechanisms of Apoptosis Induction in the CNS

Since numerous stimuli can induce apoptosis, several mechanisms have been implicated. Neuronal death after sublethal injuries, such as prolonged seizures or events in the border zone of ischemic damage, has been linked to overactivation of glutamate receptors. In turn, the resulting increase of intracellular concentrations of Ca^{2+} (Orrenius and Nicotera, 1994) can then trigger lethal biochemical pathways that involve either degrading enzymes (proteases and endonucleases) (Kerr et al., 1972; Alleva and Aloe, 1995; Pearson et al., 1995; Schreiber and Abudry, 1995) or increased synthesis of oxygen free radicals (Messmer et al., 1994). Elevated Ca^{2+} levels also induce the transcriptional activation of possibly cell death-related genes such as the immediate early genes c-jun and c-fos (Schreiber and Baudry, 1995).

Immediate-early genes, with respect to the transcriptional factors they encode, have an important function in converting extracellular signals into alterations of the cellular phenotype (Schreiber and Baudry, 1995). C-jun and c-fos may be particularly involved in the commitment to cell death. Although they are expressed transiently and at low levels in the normal brain, prolonged expression of c-fos or c-jun is associated with neuronal death (Dragnow et al., 1993). For example, c-fos is expressed during hypoxic injury of CA1 neurons in the hippocampus (Schreiber and Baudry, 1995) and c-jun expression occurs in the amygdala and the piriform cortex, both during experimentally induced seizures. The transcription factor p53 (Doussis et al., 1993; Messmer et al., 1994; Miyshito et al., 1994; Ellison et al., 1995), which also appears to possess ligase activity, functions in DNA repair mechanisms. Additionally, p53 influences the expression of c-fos (Dragnow et al., 1993) and of heat-shock protein complexes (Sharp et al., 1993) and is, therefore, likely to be associated with the commitment of a cell to apoptosis.

Proteins of the Bcl-2 family are other important factors associated with the development of apoptosis. Two homologous proteins, BCL-2 and Bcl-xl have been shown to protect cells from apoptosis (Allsopp et al., 1993; Behl et al., 1993; Boise et al., 1993; Zhong et al., 1993a,b; Akbar et al., 1994; Nunez et al., 1994; Farlie et al., 1995). Both proteins are independently capable of forming heterodimers with a third homologous protein, BAX, thus blocking it's participation in the induction of apoptosis (Oltavai et al., 1993; Miyashita et al., 1994). Bcl-2 is expressed rather abundantly in the brain during normal development (Garcia et al., 1992; Zhong et al., 1993a,b) but only at low levels in adulthood, indicating a role in the morphogenesis of the fetal brain. In contrast, bcl-x, which is probably involved in the regulation of Bcl-2 function (Boise et al., 1993) exhibits considerable expression on adult neurons Gonzalez-Garcia et al., 1995). Bcl-2 family-related mechanisms of apoptosis repression are linked to changes in intracellular Ca^{2+} influx (Lam et al., 1994).

Studies of viral infection in the brain are complicated by the fact that apoptosis and necrosis can occur simultaneously. However, viral proteins may act directly as toxic substances triggering the process of apoptosis. For example, the GP120 (Müller et al., 1992) and the tat protein of HIV (Zauli et al., 1993), p53 of baculoviruses (Messmer et al., 1994), and the gene product of herpes simplex virus g1.34.5 (Chou and Roizman, 1992) are all capable of influencing apoptosis. For example, the HIV protein GP120 acts on Ca^{2+} channels thus increasing glutamate toxicity (Müller et al., 1992; Benos et al., 1994). Additionally, in the response to viral infection, antibody-mediated cytotoxicity (Levine et al., 1991; Reid et al., 1993) and activated cytotoxic T-cells (Nishioka and Welsh, 1994) have been suggested as possible inducers of apoptosis. Cytokines secreted by T-cells or neighboring glial cells may also have a role in this process. Also demonstrated is the ability of TNF-α to induce apoptosis in the CNS (Selmaj et al., 1991), the same effect has been described for IFN-γ on cultured cerebellar granule cells (Kristensson et al., 1995). However, the role of cytokines in viral infection of the brain and in subsequent neuronal death remains unclear.

5. Detection of Apoptosis

One of the hallmarks of apoptosis is fragmentation of DNA, which is visible as "laddering" on an electrophoresis gel. However, not all forms of apoptosis appear to involve the same amount of laddering (Wyllie et al., 1984), or this phenomenon may occur at a relatively late stage in apoptosis. Additionally, this method does not allow for the identification of individual apoptotic cells. Therefore, labeling of DNA- strand breaks *in situ* is useful for identification of cells undergoing apoptosis, particularly for the detection of early stages of apoptosis. Molecular methods adapted for the detection of damaged DNA include nick translation with incorporation of digoxigenin-labeled nucleotides using DNA polymerase (Wijsman et al., 1993) and nick-end labeling with incorporation of biotin- or digoxigenin-labeled dUTP (TUNEL) using terminal deoxynucleotidyl transferase (TdT) (Gavrieli et al., 1992). These methods have proved reliable, although possibly not entirely accurate in distinguishing apoptosis from necrosis. Of the two, nick-end-labeling seems to be considerably more specific for apoptosis (Schreiber and Baudry, 1995). Nevertheless, since apoptosis must be regarded as a morphological entity, *in situ* testing for apoptosis by TUNEL requires confirmation by morphological methods.

6. Methods for Morphological Studies of Cell Death in the CNS

The following descriptions of methods for the morphological study of cell death and for TUNEL apoptosis detection focus on the use of light microscopy. However, alternative methods will be cited as well, along with references to facilitate their further evaluation.

Table 1
Fixation and Processing of Tissues for Embedding in Epoxy Resin

Step	Solutions	Time
Fixation	4% paraformaldehyde + 0.8–3% glutaraldehyde EM grade, in 0.1M sodium cacodylate buffer, pH 7.2	2 h overnight
Buffer wash	0.1M sodium cacodylate buffer	15 min overnight
Postfixation	1% aqueous osmium tetroxide (in 2–4 h fume hood)	
Wash	dest. H$_2$O	2 × 5 min
"En bloc" staining	5% aqueous uranyl acetate	30 min
Wash	dest. H$_2$O	2 × 5 min
Dehydration	50% ethanol AR grade	2 × 5 min
70% ethanol	2 × 5 min	
90% ethanol	2 × 5 min	
100% ethanol	60 min	
100% ethanol	10 min	
Clearing	propylene oxide	2 × 20 min
Resin immersion	50% epoxy resin, 50% propylene oxide	overnight
	100% epoxy resin (should be freshly made, most commercially available resins yield good results)	2 h
Embedding	in plastic capsules or rubber molds, polymerization at 60°C	1–2 d

7. Problems of Morphological Identification of Apoptosis in the CNS

In most tissues, apoptosis can be detected by light microscopy. But, because the quality of unfixed cryostat sections or those only briefly fixed is often insufficient for identifying cells with pyknosis and nuclear chromatin condensation, these minimal fixation techniques are not recommended. (For fixation procedures, *see* Tables 1 and 2.) However, formalin- or paraformaldehyde-fixed and paraffin-embedded tissues stained with hematoxylin and eosin usually provide good morphological specimens. Equally good results can be produced with Giemsa stain, which effectively differentiates nuclear structures. To the contrary, periodic acid Schiff-staining is less desirable because its dark, dense coloration fails

Table 2
Fixation and Processing of Tissues for Paraffin Embedding

Step	Solutions	Time
Fixation	4% phosphate-buffered formalin pH 7.2	24 h–6 wk
Dehydration	70% ethanol LR grade	1 × 2 h
	95% ethanol	2 × 2 h
	100% ethanol	3 × 2 h
Clearing	Xylene	2 × 2 h
Wax immersion	Paraplast wax (MP 57–58°C) at 60°C	2 × 2 h
Embedding	In molten wax	

Table 3
Stains for Light Microscopy

Stain	Solution	Procedure
Hematoxylin/ Eosin	Hematoxylin (Mayer) 2.0 g/L 0.3% Eosin Y in 70% ethanol	Hematoxylin for 15–30 s blue under running water for 5 min, then dip in eosin for 5 s, then dehydration as in Table 2
Giemsa	Giemsa: 0.8 9 Giemsa, 0.1 g Eosin Y in 100 mL 1:1 v/v glycerol and methanol buffer: 9 mL 0.1M citric acid in 25% methanol + 11 mL 0.2M Na$_2$HPO$_4$ in 25% methanol +380 mL dest. H$_2$O, pH 6.4 with HCl	Giemsa (after filtration) for 30 s–5 min, then washing in Giemsa buffer for 5 min, then dehydration as in Table 2
Methylene blue (Richardson)	1. Azur II 1% in dest. H$_2$O 2. Methylene blue 1% in 1% sodiumtetraborate. Mix both solutions 1/1 v/v	5–10 min at 60°C then washing in dest. H$_2$O for 2 min and drying at 60°C

to distinguish these structures; in fact, only extensive nuclear fragmentation becomes visible with this staining procedure. (For staining procedures, *see* Table 3). Alternatively, specific DNA stains such as acridine orange or propidium iodide

(Nicoletti et al., 1991) can be used for the detection of chromatin condensation. Sections 0.5–1 μm thick embedded in epon/araldit yield even better results, although with the disadvantage of being more time consuming than the foregoing methods. However, fragmentation of DNA is far more visible in these semithin sections than in tissue sections 5 μm or more thick embedded in paraffin, because in the latter, nuclei of apoptotic cells may appear uniformly dark.

In the CNS, recognition of apoptotic neurons is often facilitated by the slightly eosinophilic staining of their cytoplasm. However, eosinophilia may be present in necrotic cells as well, which can be distinguished from apoptotic cells by the necrosis-related swelling of cytoplasm and the disintegration of organelles. Additionally, necrosis generally appears in clusters of neighboring cells and is associated with an inflammatory process in which immune cells infiltrate the area and disrupt tissue structures. In contrast, apoptotic cells appear scattered or follow a distinct pattern of distribution. An example is the increased apoptosis in the plexus choroideus accompanying various forms of encephalitis. Apoptotic bodies derived from nuclear fragments are phagocytosed very rapidly, therefore, often are not detectable on tissue sections, or they are found in individual macrophages. However, in cell cultures where this dynamic process is not underway, a higher percentage of apoptotic bodies is likely to be detected. An additional difficulty in CNS tissue sections is that small lymphocytes infiltrating the area of interest with their dense, strongly staining nuclei can be misinterpreted as apoptotic cells. The often loose-appearing chromatin structure of astrocytes is also unfavorable to recognizing early stages of chromatin condensation. In the electron microscope, phagocytosed apoptotic bodies often lack nuclear components and may be difficult to differentiate from autophagic vacuoles, although the apoptotic bodies are usually much larger.

8. Fixation and Processing of Specimens

Fixation of brain tissue should be performed rapidly without unnecessary handling beforehand, because neuronal

staining artifacts generated by manipulation can be misinterpreted as pyknotic nuclei in neurons. When destined for
light microscopy, rodent brains may be fixed by immersion
in 4% neutrally buffered formalin or in paraformaldehyde
for 1–7 d, although previous vascular paraformaldehyde
perfusion by insertion of a butterfly infusion set (e.g., Abbott,
Dublin, Ireland) into the left heart ventricle of the deeply
anesthetized animal is preferable. If embedding in epoxy
resin is planned, the fixative should contain 4% paraformaldehyde and 3–0.08% glutaraldehyde (EM grade) in cacodylate buffer (*see* Table 1), depending on further processing of
the tissue. Since this fixative diffuses more slowly than formalin, it is advantageous to place the brains or eyes first in
4% neutrally buffered formalin for 1 d and then into a solution containing glutaraldehyde. This procedure is mandatory if whole brains are to be immersion-fixed, since nothing
less provides sufficient fixation for the entire organ. The size
of specimens placed directly into glutaraldehyde solutions
should not exceed 1–3 mm^3, and fixation time should be 1–2
d. The specimens should then be placed into cacodylate buffer
until further processing. Whole human brains are best left in
4% formalin for 5 d before sectioning or further handling.
Experimental results have demonstrated that prolonged
immersion in formalin induces a loss of immunoreactivity
for most antibodies and deterioration of TUNEL staining
(Migheli et al., 1994). However, immersion times in formalin
up to 6 wk are compatible with reproducible results for the
TUNEL technique. Tissues can be stored in paraffin indefi-
nitely without visible influence on the quality of TUNEL reactions. (For staining procedures, *see* Table 3).

Sections of paraffin-embedded tissues should be cut 3–4
µm thick and placed on poly-L-lysine-coated slides. (Alternatively, vectabond [Vector laboratories, Burlingame, CA] can
be used for coating, or sections may be placed on uncoated
superfrost+ slides [Fisher, Pittsburgh, PA] and dried at 37°C
overnight.) Deparaffination should be as complete as possible, since remaining paraffin adversely affects the TUNEL
reaction. Sections are heated at 70°C for 20 min and then

hydrated through several baths of xylene and a graded series of alcohols at concentrations ranging from 100 to 70%, with an immersion time of 3–5 min per bath.

9. The TUNEL Procedure

To expose nuclear DNA strand breaks to the enzymatic activity of TdT, sections of paraffin-embedded tissue 3–4 μm thick or sections of epoxy resin-embedded tissues 1 μm thick on slides coated as described above are treated with proteinase K. Optimal conditions include incubation for 10 min at room temperature with 20 mg/mL proteinase K in 10 mM Tris-HCl, pH 8.0. Immersion in formalin for more than a week requires higher concentrations of proteinase K and longer exposure times. However, a protease concentration of 100 mg/mL for 30 min should not be exceeded because of the ensuing morphologic deterioration. The proteinase is then washed off by rinsing with PBS four times for 3 min each. When using peroxidase-dependent detection systems, the endogenous peroxidases are inactivated by treatment with 1% H_2O_2 in methanol or 0.3% H_2O_2 in PBS. After repeated washings with PBS, the elongation of DNA fragments can begin. (For contents of buffers and reaction mix, see Table 4).

For equilibration, the slides are preincubated for up to 10 min (1 min minimum) with TdT buffer. Then the reaction mixture containing the enzyme and digoxigenin-labeled dUTP is added. The slides are incubated in a humid atmosphere for 60 min at 37°C. TdT is temperature-sensitive; temperatures above 40°C inactivate the enzyme. Depending on the size of the tissue sample, 50–100 μL of reaction mixture is allowed per section. Please note that during this reaction, drying of the sections should be avoided. Covering the sections with plastic sheets may be helpful, since this procedure not only keeps the sections from drying but also imposes an even layering of the reaction mixture over the whole tissue. (The material of most zip-lock bags has the appropriate strength for this purpose.) The reaction is terminated in a bath of basic citrate for 15–30 min at room temperature or at 37°C. After washing the slides three times in PBS, nonspe-

Table 4
TUNEL Technique for Detection of Apoptosis

Step	Solution	Procedure
Removal of parafin		70°C for 20 min
	Xylene	3 × 5 min
	100% Ethanol LR grade	3 × 5 min
	95% Ethanol	1 × 5 min
	80% Ethanol	15 × 5 min
	70% Ethanol	1 × 5 min
	PBS	1 × 5 min
Nuclear stripping	Proteinase K 20 100 µg/mL	20–30 min then wash in dest. H_2O 2 × 2 min
Blocking of endogenous peroxidases	3% H_2O_2 in methanol or 0.3% H_2O_2 in PBS	10 min then wash with PBS 2 × 3
Blocking of nonspecific reactivity	Dry nonfat milk, 5 g/L in PBS	10 min
Elongation of DNA fragments	Buffer: 30 mM trizma base, 140 mM sodium cacodylate, 1 mM cobalt chloride, pH 7.2	Preincubation 30 s–30 min at 37°C
	Reaction mix: 10X buffer as above (10% of final volume), 40–50 µM digoxigenin-dUTP, TdT 0.3 U/µL final solution, dest. H_2O	50–100 µL reaction mix per section for 60 min at 37°C
Termination	30 mM NaCl, 30 mM sodium citrate (pH 8.0)	15–30 min at room temperature or 37°C
Labeling with anti-digoxigenin peroxidase	Antidigoxigenin peroxidase dilution following manufacturers then recommendations	30 min at room temperature or at 37°C washing in PBS 3 × 5 min
Staining	DAB, 0.125 g/250 mL PBS, 1% H_2O_2	8 min at room temperature protected from light, washing in tap water for 5 min then dehydration as in Table 2

cific antigens are blocked by treatment with either 2% horse serum, 2% bovine serum albumin, or diluted nonfat dry milk (5 g/L in PBS). Slides are then incubated with antidigoxigenin-conjugated peroxidase for 30 min (100 mL per slide).

The reaction product can be visualized either with diaminobenzidine (DAB) 0.125 g/250 mL PBS (Fig. 1A) or with Vector VIP at an exposure time of 5–8 min. Light counterstaining with hematoxylin is recommended. After dehydration through increasing alcohol concentrations and several changes of xylene, the slides are mounted using an nonaqueous mounting medium (e.g., alkylacrylate). As positive controls, sections of tissues with high cellular turnover rates can be used such as those from the spleen, lymph nodes, and small intestine mucosa. High apoptosis rates are also reported for the thymic cells of dexamethasone-treated mice. However, the most stringent control for reaction conditions of this type consists of treating sections from the tissue being studied with DNAse I, which should induce DNA strand breaks and, therefore, positive reactions to TUNEL in all nuclei.

10. Alternative Staining Methods

Instead of digoxigenin-marked deoxynucleotides (dNTPs), biotin-labeled dNTPs can be used with either streptavidin-peroxidase or fluorescein-labeled avidin. Alkaline phosphatase systems yield equally good results. Performing the TUNEL reaction on epoxy resin-embedded tissues (Fig. 1B) requires a higher concentration of proteinase K (100 µg/mL for 1 h) and considerable extension of reaction times. TdT tailing should be carried out for at least 6 h. The same is valid for antidigoxigenin-peroxidase labeling. However, prior "etching" of the resin with saturated NaOH in ethanol does not improve staining results. For counterstaining of semithin sections, methylene blue has proven reliable.

A further method, similar to TUNEL although less specific for apoptosis, consists of pretreating tissues with NaSCN $1M$ at 80°C in addition to proteolytic treatment with 0.5%

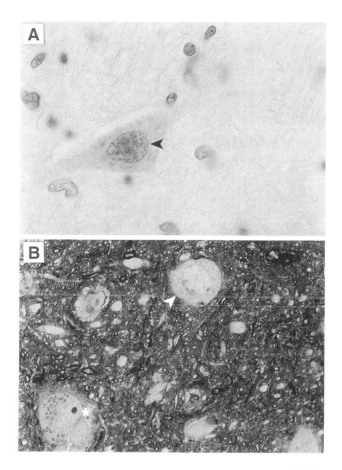

Fig. 1. TUNEL staining of neurons of brain tissue. **(A)** Detail of the gray matter within the cortex parietalis of a human brain. Note the brown DAB staining of a neuronal nucleus containing fragmented DNA. Paraffin-embedded tissue, 3 μm section, counterstaining with hematoxylin differentiated in HCl. Magnification: Orig. × 63, oil immersion. **(B)** Detail of the border zone between gray and white matter of a human brain, cortex parietalis from a patient with clinical symptoms of encephalitis. Note the loss of the nucleolus and the condensation of chromatin near the nuclear membrane, made visible by brown DAB-staining (arrow). A second neuron (asterisk) contains an intact nucleolus. Epoxy-embedded tissue, semithin cut 1 μm, counterstaining with methylene blue. Magnification: orig. × 63, oil immersion.

pepsin in HCl (pH 2.0) and using DNA polymerase I instead of TdT (Wijsman et al., 1993). This enzyme allows detection only of recessed 3' OH-DNA ends, which may be occasionally present in normal cells. In addition, it is thought that apoptotic DNA fragmentation includes the generation of DNA fragments with blunt ends and protruding ends as well (Wyllie et al., 1984). Consequently, TdT, which recognizes all forms of DNA breaks, seems to be a more suitable tool for the detection of apoptosis.

11. Comments

So far, the TUNEL technique for *in situ* localization of cells undergoing apoptosis has proven reliable and specific for differentiating this process, particularly when combined with other methods, such as DNA laddering as seen by electrophoresis (Wyllie et al., 1984) or immunocytochemistry for cell death-related antigens (Hiraishi et al., 1993), to corroborate the results. Most cells that stain positively in the TUNEL technique also show the morphological features of apoptosis, excluding other forms of cell death. However, a small number of TUNEL-positive cells, often representing smaller neurons in the brains of animals with experimental encephalitis, display apparently normal morphology. In some of these cells, electron microscopy reveals signs of nuclear damage; in a remaining small percentage, no pathology has been found. One reason for this variability may be the timing of TUNEL testing, since vislible DNA fragmentation has been regarded as a relatively late stage of apoptosis (Zakeri et al., 1993). However, we cannot entirely exclude that this notion may need revision, pointing towards an understanding of delayed cell death as a feature specific for each cell type, following a distinct timetable. As an alternative, it is possible as well that the DNA strand breaks in apparently normal cells are not beyond repair and that the cells are still viable. A further intriguing thought is that nonintegrated viral DNA (e.g., from DNA viruses like HSV), may have a role in TUNEL staining of apparently normal cells. An entirely different risk factor is that late stages of necrosis also involve fragmentation of DNA, requiring careful morphological confirmation of positive TUNEL staining.

When used with the necessary caution, the TUNEL technique represents a powerful tool for *in situ* localization of apoptotic cells and offers, therefore, a unique opportunity for studying the pathways of cell death within the CNS.

References

Akbar A. N., Salmon M., and Janossy G. (1994) Role of bcl-2 and apoptosis in viral infections. *Int. Arch. Allergy Immunol.* **105,** 359–362.

Alleva E. and Aloe L. (1995) Basic mechanisms of neuronal death: the role of nerve growth factor in neurobehavioural regulation of adult animals and humans. *J. Neuropathol. Exp. Neurol.* **54(Suppl.),** 13S.

Allsopp T. E., Wyatt S., Paterson H. F., and Davies A. M. (1993) The proto-oncogene bcl-2 can selectively rescue neurotrophic factor-dependent neurons from apoptosis. *Cell* **73,** 295–307.

Anderton B., Brion J. P., Davis D. R., and et al. (1995) Basic mechanisms of neuronal death: cytoskeletal pathology. *J. Neuropathol. Exp. Neurol.* **54(Suppl.),** 4S–5S.

Behl C., Hovey L., Krajewski S., Schubert D., and Reed J. C. (1993) Bcl-2 prevents killing of neuronal cells by glutamate but not by amyloid beta protein. *Biochem. Biophys. Res. Commun.* **197,** 949–956.

Benos D. J., Hahn B. J., Bubien J. K., Ghosh S. K., Mashourn D. A., Chaikin M. A., Shaw G. M., and Bonveniste E. N. (1994) Envelope glycoprotein gp120 of human immunodeficiency virus type 1 alters ion transport in astrocytes: implications for AIDS dementia complex. *Proc. Natl. Acad. Sci. USA* **91,** 494–498.

Boise L. H., González-Gracia M., Postema C. E., Ding L., Lindsten T., Turka L. A., Mao X., Núñez G., and Thompson C. B. (1993) Bcl-x, a bcl-2-related gene that functions as a dominant regulator of apoptotic cell death. *Cell* **74,** 597–608.

Chou J. and Roizman B. (1992) The g1 34.5 gene of herpes simplex virus 1 precludes neuroblastoma cells from triggering total shutoff of protein synthesis characteristic of programmed cell death. *Proc. Natl. Acad. Sci. USA* **89,** 3266–3207.

Doussis I. A., Pezella F., Lane D. P., Gatter K. C., and Mason D. Y. (1993) An immunocytochemical study of p53 and bcl-2 protein expression in Hodgkin's disease. *Am. J. Clin. Pathol.* **99,** 663–667.

Dragunow M., Young D., Hughes P., MacGibbon G., Lawlor P., Singleton K., Sirimanne E., Beilharc E., and Gluckman I. (1993) Is c-Jun involved in nerve cell death following status epilepticus and hypoxic-ischaemic brain injury. *Mol. Brain Res.* **18,** 347–352.

Edwards S. N., Buckmaster A. E., and Tolkovsky A. M. (1991) The death programme in cultured sympathetic neurons can be suppressed at the posttranslational level by nerve growth factor, cyclic AMP, and depoprization. *J. Neurochem.* **57,** 2140–2143.

Ellis R. E., Yuan J., and Horvitz H. R. (1991) Mechanisms and functions of cell death. *Annu. Rev. Cell Biol.* **7,** 663–689.

Ellison D. W., Lunec J., Gallagher P. J., Steart P. V., Jaros E., and Gatter K. C. (1995) Accumulation of wild type p53 in meningeomas. *Neuropathol. Appl. Neurobiol.* **21,** 136–142.

Ellison D. W., Steart P. V., Gatter K. C., and Weller R. O. (1995) Apoptosis in cerebral astrocytic tumors and its relationship to expression of the bcl-2 and p53 proteins. *Neuropathol. Appl. Neurobiol.* **21,** 352–361.

Farlie P. G., Dringen R., Rees S. M., Kannourakis G., and Bernard O. (1995) Bcl-2 transgene expression can protect neurons against developmental and induced cell death. *Proc. Natl. Acad. Sci. USA* **92,** 4397–4401.

Ferrer I., Martin F., Serrano T., Reiriz J., Pérez-Navarro E., Alberch J., Macaya A., and Planas A. M. (1995) Both apoptosis and necrosis occur following intrastriatal administration of excitotoxins. *Acta Neuropathol. Berl.* **90,** 504–510.

Fluckiger A. C., Durand I., and Banchereau J. (1994) Interleukin 10 induces apoptotic cell death of B-chronic lymphocytic leukemia cells. *J. Exp. Med.* **179,** 91–99.

Forloni G. C. R., Smiroldo S., Verga L., Salmona M., Tagliavini F., and Angeretti N. (1993) Apoptosis mediated neurotoxicity induced by chronic application of b amyloid fragment 25–35. *NeuroReport* **4,** 523–526.

Freeman S. M., Abboud C. N., Whartenby K. A., Packman C. H., Koeplin D. S., and Moolten F. L. (1993) The "bystander effect" tumor regression when a fraction of the tumor mass is genetically modified. *Cancer Res.* **53,** 5274–5283.

Garcia I., Martinou I., Tsujimoto Y., and Martinou J. C. (1992) Prevention of programmed cell death of sympathetic neurons by the bcl-2 proto-oncogene. *Science* **258,** 302–304.

Gavrieli Y., Sherman Y., and Ben-Sasson S. A. (1992) Identification of programmed cell death in situ via specific labeling of nuclear DNA fragmentation. *J. Cell Biol.* **119,** 493–501.

Geiger K. D., Deepak G., Howes E. L., Lewandowski G. A., Reed J. C., Bloom F. E., and Savvetnick N. E. (1995) Cytokine-mediated survival from lethal herpes simplex virus-infection: role of programmed neuronal death. *Proc. Natl. Acad. Sci. USA* **92,** 3411–3415.

Giese A. H. G. M. and Hess B. (1995) Neuronal cell death in scrapie-infected mice is due to apoptosis. *Brain Pathol.* **5,** 213–221.

Gonzáles-Garcia M., Garcia I., Ding L., O'Shea S., Boise L. H., Thompson C. B., and Núñez G. (1995) bcl-x is expressed in embryonic and postnatal neural tissues and functions to prevent neuronal cell death. *Proc. Natl. Acad. Sci. USA* **92,** 4304–4308.

Griffin D. E., Levine B., Tyor W. R., Tucker P. C., and Hardwick J. M. (1994) Age-dependent susceptibility to fatal encephalitis: alphavirus infection of neurons. *Arch. Virol.* **9(Suppl.),** 31–39.

Hiraishi K., Suzuki K., Hakomori S., and Adachi M. (1993) Ley antigen expression is correlated with apoptosis (programmed cell death). *Glycobiology* **3,** 381–390.

Jeffrey M., Fraser J. R., Halliday W. G., Fowler N., Goodsir C. M., and Brown D. A. (1995) Early unsuspected neuron and axon terminal loss in scrapie-infected mice revealed by morphometry and immunocytochemistry. *Neuropathol. Appl. Neurobiol.* **21,** 41–49.

Kerr J. F. R., Searle J., Harmon B. V., and Bishop C. J. (1987) Apoptosis, in *Perspectives on Mammalian Cell Death.* Potton C. S., ed. Oxford University Press, Oxford, UK, pp. 93–128.

Kerr J. F. R., Wyllie A. H., and Currie A. R. (1972) Apoptosis, a basic biological phenomenon with wide-ranging implication in tissue kinetics. *Br. J. Cancer* **26,** 239–257.

Kornbluth R. S. (1994) The immunological potential of apoptotic debris produced by tumor cells and during HIV infection. *Immunol. Lett.* **43,** 125–132.

Kristensson K., Diana A., and Nicotera P. (1995) Interferon-gamma-induced apoptosis in cerebellar granular cells. 25th Annual conference of the Society for *Neuroscience.* San Diego, CA, Society for *Neuroscience* **2(1),** 1.

Lam M., Dubyak G., Chen L., Nunez G., Miesfeld R. L., Distelhorst C. W. (1994) Evidence that BCL-2 represses apoptosis by regulating endoplasmic reticulum-associated Ca2+ fluxes. *Proc. Natl. Acad. Sci. USA* **91,** 6569–6573.

Lassmann H., Bancher C., Breitschopf H., et al. (1995) Cell death in Alzheimer's disease evaluated by DNA fragmentation in situ. *Acta Neuropathol.* **89,** 35–41.

Levine B., Hardwick J. M., Trapp B. D., Crawford T. O., Bollinger R. C., and Griffin D. E. (1991) Antibody-mediated clearance of alphavirus infection from neurons. *Science* **254,** 856–560.

Mangan D. F., Robertson B., and Wahl S. M. (1992) Il-4 enhances programmed cell death (apoptosis) in stimulated human monocytes. *J. Immunol.* **148,** 1812–1816.

Messmer U. K., Ancarcrona M., Nicotera P., and Brune B. (1994) p53 expression in nitric oxide-induced apoptosis. *FEBS Lett.* **355,** 23–26.

Migheli A., Cavalla P., Marino S., and Schiffer D. (1994) A study of apoptosis in normal and pathologic nervous tissue after in situ end-labeling of DNA strand breaks. *J. Neuropathol. Exp. Neurol.* **53,** 606–616.

Miyashita T., Krajewski S., Krajewska M., Wang H. G., Lin H. K., Liebermann D. A., Hoffman B., and Reed J. C. (1994) Tumor suppressor p53 is a regulator of bcl-2 and bax gene expression in vitro and in vivo. *Oncogene* **9**, 1799–1805.

Mochizuki H., Nakamura N., Nishi K., and Mizuno Y. (1994) Apoptosis is induced by 1-methyl-4-pyridinium ion (MPP+) in ventral mesencephalic-striatal co-culture in rat. *Neurosci. Lett.* **170**, 191–194.

Müller W. E., Schröder H. C., Ushijima H., Dapper J., and Bormann J. (1992) gp120 of HIV-1 induces apoptosis in rat cortical cell cultures: prevention by memantine. *Eur. J. Pharmacol.* **226**, 209–214.

Nicoletti I., Migliorati G., Pagliacci M. C., Grignani F., and Riccardi C. (1991) A rapid and simple method for measuring thymocyte apoptosis by propidium iodide staining and flow cytometry. *J. Immunol. Methods* **139**, 271–279.

Nishioka W. K. and Welsh R. M. (1994) Susceptipility to cytotoxic T lymphocyte-induced apoptosis is a function of the proliferative status of the target. *J. Exp. Med.* **179**, 769–774.

Nunez G., Merino R., Grillot D., and Gonzales-Garcia M. (1994) Bcl-2 and Bcl-x: regulatory switches for lymphoid death and survival. *Immunol. Today* **15**, 582–588.

Oltavai Z. N., Milliman C. L., and Korsmeye S. J. (1993) Bcl-2 heterodimerizes in vivo with a conserved homolog, Bax, that accelerates programmed cell death. *Cell* **74**, 609–619.

Oppenheim R. W., Houenou L. J., Johnson J. E., et al. (1995) Developing motor neurons rescued from programmed and axotomy-induced cell death by GDNF. *Nature* **373**, 344–346.

Orrenius S. and Nicotera P. (1994) The calcium ion and cell death. *J. Neurol. Transm.* **43(Suppl.)**, 1–11.

Pearson S. J., Sardar A. M., and Eggett C. J. (1995) Basic mechanisms of neuronal death: excitatory neurotoxicity and its role in neurodegeneration disease processes. *J. Neuropathol. Exp. Neurol.* **54(Suppl.)**, 10S,11S.

Pittman R. N., Mills J. C., DiBenedetto A. J., Hynicka W. P., and Wang S. (1994) Neuronal cell death: searching for the smoking gun. *Curr. Opinion Neurobiol.* **4**, 87–94.

Reid D. M., Perry V. H., Andersson P. B., and Gordon S. (1993) Mitosis and apoptosis of microglia in vivo induced by an anti CR3 antibody which crosses the blood-brain barrier. *Neuroscience* **56**, 529–533.

Schreiber S. S. and Baudry M. (1995) Selective neuronal vulnerability in the hippocampus-a role for gene expression. *Trends Neurosci.* **18**, 446–451.

Selmaj K., Raine C. S., Faroq M., Norton W. T., and Brosnan C. F. (1991) Cytokine cytotoxicity against oligodendrocytes. Apoptosis induced by lymphotoxin. *J. Immunol.* **147**, 1522–1529.

Sharp F. R., Kinouch H., Koistinaho J., Chan P. K., and Sagar S. M. (1993) HSP70 heat shock gene regulation during ischemia. *Stroke* **24(Suppl. 1)**, I.72–I.75.

Ubol S., Tucker P. C., Griffin D. E., and Hardwick J. M. (1994) Neurovirulent strains of alphavirus induce apoptosis in bcl-2-expressing cells: role of a single amino acid change in the E2 glycoprotein. *Proc. Natl. Acad. Sci. USA* **91**, 5202–5206.

Walkinshaw G. and Waters C. M. (1994) Neurotoxin-induced cell death in neuronal PC12 cells is mediated by induction of apoptosis. *Neuroscience* **63**, 975–987.

Wijsman J. H., Jonker R. R., Keijzer R., Van de Velde C. J. H., Cornelisse C. J., and Va Dierenconck J. H. (1993) A new method to detect apoptosis in paraffin sections: in situ end-labeling of fragmented DNA. *J. Histochem. Cytochem.* **42**, 7–12.

Wyllie A. H. (1980) Glucocorticoid-induced thymocyte apoptosis is associated with endogenous endonuclease activation. *Nature* **284**, 555,556.

Wyllie A. H., Morris R. G., Smith A. L., and Dunlop D. (1984) Chromatin cleavage in apoptosis: association with condensed chromatin morphology and dependence on macromolecular synthesis. *J. Pathol.* **142**, 67–77.

Yoshiyama Y., Yamada T., Asanuma K., and Asahi T. (1994) Apoptosis-related antigen Le(Y) and nick-end labeling are positive in spinal motorneurons in amyotrophic lateral sclerosis. *Acta Neuropathol.* **88**, 207–211.

Zakeri Z. F., Quaglino D., Latham T., and Lockshin R. A. (1993) Delayed internucleosomal DNA-fragmentation in programmed cell death. *FASEB J.* **7**, 470–478.

Zauli G., Gibellini D., Milani D., Mazzoni M., Borgatti P., La Placa M., and Capitani S. (1993) Human immunodeficiency virus type-1 Tat protein protects lymphoid, epithelial, and neuronal cell lines from death by apoptosis. *Cancer Res.* **53**, 4481–4485.

Zhong L. T., Kane D. J., and Bredesen D. E. (1993a) BCL-2 blocks glutamate toxicity in neural cell lines. *Brain Res.* **19**, 353–355.

Zhong L. T., Sarafian T., Kane D. J., Charles A. C., Hah S. P., Edwards R. H., and Bredesen D. E. (1993b) bcl-2 inhibits death of central neural cells induced by multiple agents. *Proc. Natl. Acad. Sci. USA* **90**, 4533–4537.

Techniques for Distinguishing Apoptosis from Necrosis in Cerebrocortical and Cerebellar Neurons

Emanuela Bonfoco, Maria Ankarcrona, Dimitri Krainc, Pierluigi Nicotera, and Stuart A. Lipton

1. Introduction

Apoptosis is a form of regulated cell death, characterized by a series of morphological alterations including cell shrinkage, chromatin condensation, pyknosis of the nucleus, and multistep chromatin degradation (*see* references in Bonfoco et al., 1995 and in Ankarcrona et al., 1995). The latter includes the cleavage of DNA into high (700–50 kbp) and low (oligonucleosomal) fragments. Despite the exponential growth of research on apoptosis during the past few years, the detection of this form of cell death both in vitro and in vivo has primarily relied on morphological criteria. Thus, electron and light microscopy have been the techniques of choice to identify apoptotic cells. Nevertheless, detection of apoptosis based on purely morphological criteria has some limitations. It cannot be utilized to efficiently screen large numbers of samples. Further, it is becoming increasingly clear that different cell types may adopt different morphological patterns of involution, and even the same cell type may vary in appearance in response to disparate apoptotic stimuli. For example, the morphological appearance of immature T-lym-

From: *Neuromethods, Vol. 29: Apoptosis Techniques and Protocols*
Ed: J. Poirier Humana Press Inc.

phocytes undergoing apoptosis after treatment with dexamethasone differs from that of T-cells killed by FAS/APO1. Neurons, at least in culture, often remain adherent to the dish, displaying apoptotic condensed nuclei (Deckwerth and Johnson, 1994; Ankarcrona et al., 1995). In contrast, individual cells in dividing cell lines tend to loose adherence, condense, and detach from the dish. In contrast, endothelial cells appear to undergo condensation of chromatin and become typically apoptotic only after detachment.

The literature concerning the issue of whether a neuronal cell population will or will not undergo apoptosis has been complicated by the tendency of many authors to rely on a single criterion (i.e., DNA laddering, sensitivity to inhibitors of protein synthesis, and so on). As we have recently proposed (Bonfoco et al., 1995; Ankarcrona et al., 1995), it is mandatory to use multiple rather than single end-points to avoid misinterpretation of data suggestive of apoptosis vs necrosis.

In this chapter, we describe short protocols used in our laboratories to detect apoptosis in neuronal cell cultures and in tissue samples.

2. Morphological Detection of Apoptosis and Necrosis in Neuronal Cultures

2.1. Use of Fluorescent Nuclear Dyes

Apoptotic cells characteristically condense and eventually fragment their nuclei prior to plasma membrane damage. Formation of membrane enclosed apoptotic nuclei is the single criterion that is most utilized to indicate the presence of apoptosis. Because of this characteristic, the combination of cell permeant and impermeant nuclear dyes can provide information on the fate of the neuron in cell culture. We have recently used a combination of two fluorescent nuclear stains available from Molecular Probes (Eugene, OR): propidium iodide and SYTO-13. Propidium iodide is a well-known nuclear stain that binds DNA with little or no base pair preference. It can be excited by a Krypton argon laser (488–547 nm), and the resulting emission can be collected in the red wavelengths of the spectrum. On DNA or RNA binding, propidium iodide fluorescence is enhanced. Propidium iodide is excluded from cells that retain membrane integrity, including viable neurons and neurons that already have developed apoptotic nuclei (Ankarcrona et al., 1995). In contrast, SYTO-13, one of the latest generation of membrane-permeant nuclear probes, will stain the nuclei of viable cells green. Thus, when cells preloaded with SYTO-13 are exposed to a medium containing propidium iodide, necrotic cells (i.e., cells with compromised or lysed plasma membranes) will stain progressively yellow (the combination of red and green) and then red, as the propidium gains access to the DNA. On the other hand, viable cells will retain the green staining as well as their normal nuclear size and appearance. Neurons undergoing necrosis will display normal or slightly large nuclei that are stained by propidium iodide, whereas debris of genetic material may diffuse into the culture medium from frankly necrotic neurons with lysed membranes. Conversely, the nuclei of apoptotic neurons will exclude the red propidium iodide (unless they have been vigorously permeabdilized by detergent) and, instead, will retain the green SYTO-13 fluorescence in pyknotic (small) nuclei with condensed chromatin. Using this technique, we have been able to elucidate a sequence of necrosis followed by apoptosis in different populations of cerebellar granule cell neurons exposed to glutamate (Fig. 1) (Ankarcrona et al., 1995).

2.2. Methods for Fluorescent Nuclear Dyes in Unpermeabilized Neurons

Neurons grown on coverslips are first loaded with SYTO-13 (0.5 μM) for 20 min at 37°C in culture medium containing 2% fetal bovine serum (loading is more efficient in buffers with low phosphate; however, in the experimental systems we used, loading was sufficient also in the presence of normal phosphate concentrations). Coverslips are subsequently placed under the (preferably confocal) microscope in an incubation chamber and superfused with incubation buffer containing propidium iodide (10 µg/mL). Cells can be treated

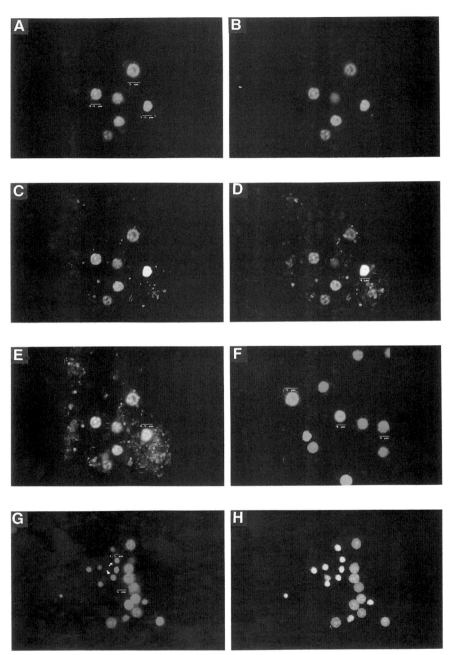

Fig. 1.

in a perfusion chamber directly under the microscope or preexposed to propidium iodide and subsequently loaded with SYTO-13. Fluorescence is then collected in the green and red ranges. Using a confocal microscope with a suitable image analysis system, nuclear diameters can be calculated, and apoptotic or necrotic cells can be scored for a quantitative estimation (Ankarcrona et al., 1995).

Fig. 1. *(previous page)* Necrosis and apoptosis of cerebellar granule cells stimulated by glutamate. **(A–E)** Neurons were loaded with 0.5 μM SYTO-13 and exposed to glutamate in the presence of propidium iodide (10 μg/mL). Neurons that died by necrosis progressively exhibited a fluorescence shift from green to orange-red because propidium iodide gained entry into the nucleus. Nuclei did not become pyknotic. Instead, they swelled and then fragmented, spreading genetic material (stained in red by propidium iodide) into the surrounding medium. (A) Control. (B) After a 3-mM glutamate exposure of 7 min duration, (C) 10 min duration, (D) 15 min duration, and (E) 30 min duration. In the field illustrated in (A–E), a single neuron developed propidium iodide staining. The diameter of the nucleus increased from 3.6 μm under control conditions to 4.5 μm. Simultaneously, red debris appeared from the neurons just outside of the field that had also undergone necrosis. **(F)** Another field after a 30 min exposure to glutamate followed by a wash to remove debris. The number of neurons stained by propidium iodide in this manner was counted in 10 fields in three separate experiments (more than 400 neurons scored). After a 30 min exposure to 3 mM glutamate, a significant member of neurons underwent necrosis (38 ± 4%; mean ± SD; $p < 0.05$ by Student's t-test). **(G, H)** Cerebellar granule cells surviving early glutamate exposure undergo delayed nuclear condensation typical of apoptosis. Neurons loaded with SYTO-13 were imaged 6 h after exposure to glutamate. Propidium iodide (10 μg/mL) was included in the incubation medium. (G) Apparently normal neurons had larger nuclear diameters than apoptotic nuclei, which also lacked discernible chromatin structure. Normal nuclei in this experiment had diameters of 3.8 ± 0.6 μm (mean ± SD, $n = 30$). Apoptotic nuclei were significantly smaller, averaging 1.7 ± 0.2 μm ($n = 30$; $p < 0.05$ by Student's t-test). (H) Permeabilization with high concentrations of Triton X-100 (10%) produced partial staining of apoptotic nuclei with propidium iodide (shift toward yellow-orange fluorescence) and complete staining of apparently normal nuclei (red fluorescence). Reproduced with permission from Ankarcrona et al. (1995). For color photographs, please see the original article.

2.3. Methods for Fluorescent Nuclear Dyes
in Permeabilized Neurons

Staining with propidium iodide can also be very useful in revealing details of chromatin structural changes in samples that are fixed and *permeabilized*. Other dyes may also be used for this purpose, such as Hoechst 33258. Neurons on glass coverslips are gently rinsed two times with phosphate-buffered saline (PBS) and then fixed and permeabilized with methanol:water (4:1) 15 min. After rinsing with PBS, the coverslips are stained with propidium iodide (5 µg/mL) for 5 min in the dark and mounted on glass slides in glycerol:PBS (1: 1). Instead of propidium iodide, Hoechst dye 33528 (2.5 µg/mL) can be used to assess apoptosis by nuclear staining (blue) after fixation of cells in paraformaldehyde (4%). The glass slides are preferentially examined under confocal laser scanning microscopy. Apoptotic nuclei are hyperfluorescent, condensed or fragmented, and smaller compared to normal nuclei as shown in Fig. 2. The nuclear hyperfluorescence and the nuclear size change can be utilized with appropriate video-image analysis systems to provide a semi-automatic scoring system for apoptotic cells.

2.4. Electron Microscopy

Electron microscopy remains the most reliable method of characterizing apoptotic features both in tissue sections and in cell culture. Images of condensed nuclei with nuclear margination, blebbing, and typical shrinkage of the cytoplasm are diagnostic of apoptosis. Mitochondria appear intact (i.e., with no apparent sign of swelling) although an aggregation of mitochondria around the nucleus has been observed in some cells. Vacuolization of the cytoplasm is usually absent from typical apoptotic cells; membranes appear intact, at least in the early stages.

Care in the interpretation of the data should be exercised when a mixture of apoptotic and necrotic features are seen in the same sample. It is now clear that secondary necrosis may occur when the ability to remove apoptotic cells by phagocytes is insufficient or compromised, and this is common

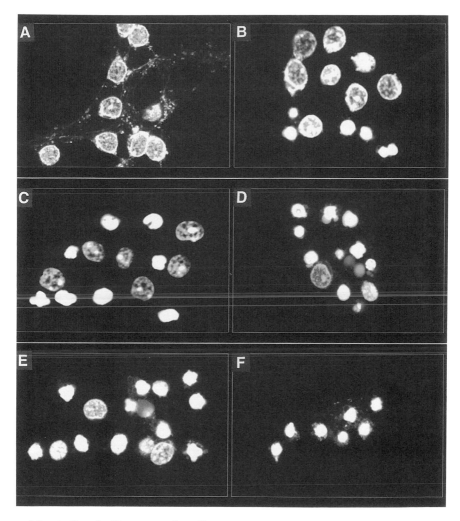

Fig. 2. Cerebellar granule cell neurons exposed to glutamate undergo chromatin condensation. Neurons were exposed to various concentrations of glutamate for 30 min and then incubated in culture medium for the times indicated below. The cultures were then fixed, permeabilized, stained with propidium iodide, and examined by confocal microscopy. **(A)** Control at 24 h, **(B)** 30 µM glutamate at 24 h, **(C)** 100 µM glutamate at 24 h, **(D)** 3 mM glutamate at 6 h, **(E)** 3 mM glutamate at 9 h, and **(F)** 3 mM glutamate at 12 h. Note that in (B) and (D) some preapoptotic nuclei exhibiting chromatin buttoning can be seen near typically condensed nucilei.

under tissue culture conditions. It is not infrequent, therefore, to observe cells with apoptotic, fragmented nuclei and secondary plasma membrane lysis. Additionally, however, the same insult can lead to temporally distinct phases of apoptosis and necrosis. For example, we found that mild insults with glutamate or nitric oxide/superoxide to cerebrocortical neurons in vitro led to apoptosis of delayed onset, whereas intense exposure led to more rapid necrosis within a few hours (Bonfoco et al., 1995). For cerebellar granule cell neurons in culture, we found that exposure to glutamate induced a wave of necrosis in a subpopulation of the cells, followed by delayed apoptosis in another subpopulation (Ankarcrona et al., 1995). The methodology to observe apoptotic vs necrotic morphology at the ultrastructural level is comprised of the typical sample fixation used for other applications of electron microscopy.

2.5. Methods for Electron Microscopy

Tissue samples or cultures are fixed in 1% glutaraldehyde diluted in 0.1M phosphate buffer, at pH 7.2 (Yun and Kenney, 1976). The tissue is cut in 1-μm slices and fixed for 5 h at room temperature and than postfixed with 1% osmium tetroxide in PBS for 1 h. After dehydrating samples in acetone and embedding them in epon, thin sections are cut on a LKB ultratome, counterstained with uranyl acetate, and examined with an electron microscope.

3. Analysis of DNA Fragmentation on Agarose Gels

The cleavage of DNA into oligonucleosomes reflects the organized degradation of chromatin during the apoptotic process. DNA fragmentation into oligonucleosomal length fragments has been extensively used as the most reliable biochemical marker for apoptosis (Wyllie, 1980; Arends and Wyllie, 1991). In many papers in the literature, the resulting laddering pattern on 1.0–1.5% agarose gels has often been the single criterion used to determine the occurrence of apoptosis. However, more recent work has shown that DNA laddering is a rather late event in the apoptotic process

(Brown et al., 1993; Oberhammer et al., 1993; Zhivotovsky et al., 1994). Apoptotic nuclei can, in fact, form before the appearance of oligonucleosomal fragmentation. Thus, whereas the presence of DNA laddering is typical for apoptosis (and no strong evidence has been provided for its occurrence in necrotic cell death), the absence of oligonucleosomal fragmentation cannot be used to exclude apoptosis in neurons (Ankarcrona et al., 1995). The formation of larger chromatin fragments (i.e., 50 kbp) correlates more closely with the appearance of apoptotic nuclei. The nature of these fragments is still unclear. It has been proposed that 50 kbp fragments may represent single chromatin loops, whereas larger fragments (300 kbp) may be aggregates of multiple loops, representing rosettes.

Formation of high-mol-wt DNA fragments can be detected by field inversion gel electrophoresis (FIGE), whereas oligonucleosomal fragmentation is traditionally demonstrated by conventional agarose gel electrophoresis. An elegant combination of the two techniques, involving the recovery of small fragments from the plugs used for the FIGE, allows for the simultaneous detection of both high and low-mol-wt DNA fragments. Oligonucleosomal fragmentation can also be measured semiquantitatively using an enzyme-linked immunoadsorbent assay (ELISA) to detect immunocomplexes of antibodies reacting with nucleosomes. Finally, morphological detection of DNA nicks can also be performed on tissue sections or on cultured cells using a nick-end labeling procedure known as the TUNEL technique (TdT-mediated dUTP-biotin nick-end labeling).

3.1. Methods for Gel Electrophoresis of DNA

3.1.1. Field Inversion Gel Electrophoresis (FIGE)

Neurons are gently removed from culture dishes and suspended in a solution containing $0.15M$ NaCl, 2 mM KH_2PO_4, pH 6.8, 1 mM EGTA, and 5 mM $MgCl_2$. An equal volume of liquefied 1% low melting point agarose gel solution is then added to the suspension, while gently mixing. Next, the mixture is aliquoted into gel plug casting forms and allowed to cool and solidify on ice for 10 min. The resulting agarose blocks are transferred into a solution containing 10 mM NaCl, 10 mM Tris-HCl, pH 9.5, 25 mM EDTA, 1% lauroylsarcosine, and 200 µg/mL proteinase K, and incubated for 24 h at 50°C with continuous agitation. The plugs are then rinsed three times over 24 h at 4°C in 10 mM Tris-HCl, pH 8.0, and 1 mM EDTA. Subsequently, the plugs are stored until used for electrophoresis at 4°C in 50 mM EDTA, pH 8.0. FIGE is performed with horizontal or vertical gel chambers. We currently use horizontal gel chambers (HE100B) and a switchback pulse controller (PC 500, Hoefer Scientific, San Francisco, CA) equipped with a constant temperature cooling system. The temperature control is very important. Normally, we run the electrophoresis at 180 V in 1% agarose gel in 0.5 TBE (45 mM Tris, 1.25 mM EDTA, 45 mM boric acid, pH 8.0) at 12°C. The ramp rate changes from 20–30 s for the first 6 h, 10–20 s for the second 6 h, and 0.8–10 s for the next 12 h, applying a forward to reverse ratio of 3:1 (Ankarcrona et al., 1995).

3.1.2. Conventional Agarose Gels

Neurons (1 × 10^7) are lysed at room temperature for 60 min in a buffer containing 0.5% Triton X-100, 5 mM Tris-buffer, pH 7.4, and 20 mM EDTA. The lysate is than incubated with proteinase K (100 µg/mL) for 2 h at 37°C. Following RNAse treatment for 1 h at 37°C, DNA is extracted with an equal volume of phenol/chloroform (1:1) and precipitated with 1/10 vol 7M ammonium acetate and 2.5 vol ice-cold ethanol at room temperature or –20°C for 1 h. After centrifugation at 14,000g, the DNA pellets are resuspended in distilled water and loaded onto a 1.4% agarose gel. The gel electrophoresis is run at 90 V for approx 2 h (Wyllie et al., 1980). Alternatively, DNA fragmentation in oligonucleosomal fragments can be detected by collecting the DNA released from the agarose plugs during the incubation with proteinase. This fraction is precipitated with 2 vol of absolute ethanol in the presence of 5M NaCl. The DNA is subsequently loaded onto conventional 1.8% agarose gels and run as described above.

4. *In Situ* Labeling of Nuclear DNA Fragments

The TUNEL technique is a method to visualize strand breaks in DNA and can be applied to both tissue sections and cell cultures (Gavrieli et al., 1992). It is commonly used to detect DNA damage and therefore apoptotic cells. The principle of this technique is based on the addition of dUDP-biotin to the end nicks of strand breaks using a reaction catalyzed by terminal transferase. A secondary reaction with antibodies or other detection systems is used to detect the nicks. With the TUNEL technique it is possible to discriminate morphologically the apoptotic nuclei by the presence of strand breaks in the DNA (evidenced by labeling the nicked ends of DNA) from areas of labeled necrotic cells, in which random DNA degradation occurs. However, any random DNA cleavage can eventually expose a 3'OH strand break that can potentially be labeled by the TUNEL technique. This may or may not be detected, but, in any event, it is the coexistence of TUNEL positivity with the aforementioned morphological changes, including condensed pyknotic nuclei, that demonstrates apoptosis. One must be aware that the potential pitfall of the TUNEL technique is that necrotic cells may sometimes appear positive as a result of random DNA cleavage.

4.1. Methods for the TUNEL Technique

Neurons are permeabilized and fixed with 80% methanol for 15 min and then incubated with 2% hydrogen peroxide for 5 mm at room temperature to decrease endogenous peroxidase activity. This step is omitted when staining is achieved using fluorescent antibodies. The samples are then incubated with terminal deoxynucleotidyl transferase (0.3 U/µL) and biotinylated dUTP (40 µM) for 1 h at 37°C. Subsequently, neurons are exposed to extra-avidin peroxidase for 30 min at 37°C. Staining with 3-3'dimaminobenzidine (DAB) follows for 3–5 min at room temperature. Alternatively, staining with avidin-conjugated fluorescent antibodies can be used for detection by a microscope equipped for epifluorescence. The TUNEL technique always requires positive controls using DNase treatment (1 μg/mL) to create artificial nicks in the chromatin in a given preparation.

5. Cell Death Detection ELISA

As discussed above, mono- and oligonucleosomal fragmentation can be a feature of cells undergoing apoptosis, including neurons. The detection of DNA laddering is often problematic when only a few cells in the population undergo apoptosis. A more sensitive detection of oligonucleosomal fragmentation can be performed using a sandwich-enzyme immunoassay that uses mouse MAbs directed against DNA and histones. This provides a quantitative in vitro determination of histone-associated DNA fragments (mono-oligonucleosomes) in the cytoplasmic fraction of cell lysates. Thus, the ELISA uses MAbs to detect an increase in histone proteins that is associated with the fragmented DNA of the mono- and oligonucleosomes observed in the cytoplasm of apoptotic neurons (Bonfoco et al., 1995).

5.1. Methods for ELISA in the Analysis of Apoptosis

In the first step, antihistone MAbs are absorbed to the bottom of a microtiter plate. Subsequently, nonspecific binding sites are saturated by incubation with a blocking solution. A second incubation follows, wherein the nucleosomes contained in the tissue samples bind via their histone components to the immobilized antihistone antibodies. Finally, in a third incubation, anti-DNA peroxidase reacts with the DNA component of the nucleosome. Immunocomplexes can be detected spectrophotometrically with an ELISA plate reader at 405 nm. This ELISA to quantify apoptosis is available commercially as a kit (Boehringer Mannheim, Mannheim, Germany, cat. no. 1544 675).

6. Measurements of Mitochondrial Membrane Potential

Recent studies in our laboratories as well as in others have indicated that mitochondrial function can be important in determining whether a cell will die by apoptosis or necrosis. We studied cerebellar granule cell neurons in culture and found that glutamate-induced collapse of mitochondrial membrane potential accompanied by generalized energy loss leads to rapid mitochondrial and neuronal swelling followed by necrotic cell death (Ankarcrona et al., 1995). In contrast, neurons that recover mitochondrial membrane potential and near-normal function progress subsequently to an apoptotlc program of cell death. To visualize changes in the mitochondrial membrane potential in cerebellar granule cells, we used the fluorescent probe 5,5',6,6'-tetrachloro-1,1',3,3'-tetraethyl-benzimidazolocarbocyanide iodide (JC-1, Molecular Probes). JC-1 is a lipophilic carbocyanide with a delocalized positive charge. Its uptake is driven by the membrane potential, which is negative inside energized mitochondria. Depending on the mitochondrial membrane potential, JC-1 forms aggregates (termed J-aggregates) and undergoes a reversible shift in emission from 527 nm (green fluorescence) to 590 nm (red fluorescence) as more J-aggregates form at increasingly negative (hyperpolarized) mitochondrial potentials.

In primary cerebellar granule cell cultures, depolarization of the mitochondrial membrane potential occurs very rapidly during exposure to glutamate. Conversion of red to green fluorescence (loss of J-aggregates) reflects depolarization of the membrane potential; loss of both green and red fluorescence is indicative of cell permeabilization, leakage of the dye, and thus necrosis (Fig. 3) (Ankarcrona et al., 1995).

6.1. Methods for the Use
of Mitochondrial Membrane Potential-Sensing Dyes

Neurons grown on poly-L-lysine coated coverslips are loaded with JC-1 dye (1.0 μg/mL) for 30 min at 37°C in culture medium containing 2% fetal bovine serum. The neurons are then placed under a confocal microscope and superfused with the buffer of choice (in our experiments with glutamate exposure of rat cerebellar granule cells, we used nominally Mg^{2+}-free Locke-25 medium supplemented with glycine). JC-1 is excited at 488 nm and fluorescence emission is monitored

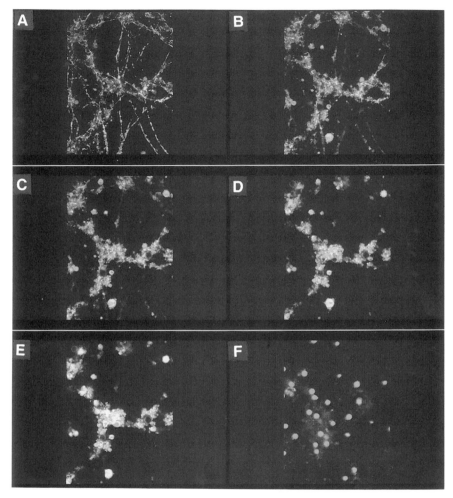

Fig. 3. Glutamate induces loss of mitochondrial membrane potential in cerebellar granule cell neurons. Neurons were loaded with JC-1
as described in the text. The dye is not retained by cells that become
permeabilized. **(A)** Before the addition of glutamate, peripheral mitochondria fluoresced red, indicating a hyperpolarized membrane
potential, whereas mitochondria in cell somas and some processes
stained green, indicating more depolarized potentials. **(B–D)** Neurons
were exposed to 3 m*M* glutamate, and images were collected with a
confocal microscope at 10, 15, and 30 min. **(E)** Glutamate was washed
out, and neurons were superfused with medium containing propidium
iodide (10 µg/mL). Cells with damaged membranes lost their JC-1

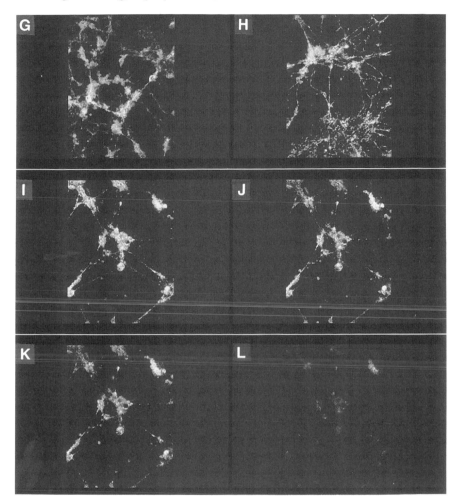

fluorescence and took up propidium iodide, yielding a red fluorescence.
(F) After addition of Triton X-100 (0.5%), all neurons were permeabilized
and stained red by propidium iodide. The JC-1 staining disappeared on
permeabilization. **(G)** Another group of neurons was exposed to glutamate
for 30 min. **(H)** Subsequent wash for 30 min resulted in restoration of the
mitochondrial membrane potential, shown by the presence of many
processes exhibiting red fluorescence. **(I–L)** Readdition of 3 m*M* glutamate
again caused a loss JC-1 fluorescence, illustrated immediately after
exposure to glutamate and at 5, 10, and 15 min. Reproduced with permission from Ankarcrona et al. (1995). For color photographs, please see the
original article.

at green and red wavelengths. Short exposures to laser light are recommended to minimize photobleaching of the fluorescent probe. Qualitative information on mitochondrial membrane potential can be derived from the shift from red to green fluorescence, indicating depolarization of the mitcochondrial membrane potential, or from the loss of fluorescence caused by neuronal cell lysis. In addition, the ratio of red and green fluorescence can be used to obtain quantitative analyses.

7. Concluding Remarks

Here we describe several criteria that are distinctive for apoptosis in neurons. These include morphological criteria using fluorescent nuclear dyes or electron microscopy, analysis of DNA fragmentation on agarose gels, *in situ* labeling of nuclear DNA fragments, ELISA of histone-associated DNA fragments (mono- and oligonucleosomes), and measurements of mitochondrial membrane potential.

We also emphasize that there are several potential pitfalls in distinguishing apoptosis from necrosis in neurons (or other cell types for that matter). Chief among these are the following:

1. The recognition that similar stimuli can result in either apoptosis or necrosis, depending on the intensity of the initial insult.
2. The fact that secondary necrosis can eventually develop if phagocytes do not eliminate the apoptotic cells.
3. Several criteria must be used to define features of apoptosis, as any one criteria may be misleading under certain conditions.
4. The TUNEL and related techniques in particular may result in misleading results if other criteria are not used in conjunction, such as the presence of pyknotic nuclei.

Distinguishing necrosis from apoptosis in neurons in various neurodegenerative disorders may help in the elucidation of the underlying pathogenic mechanism of each disease and may thus have therapeutic implications (Lipton and Rosenberg, 1994). In the future, it will be important to determine the molecular events and signal transduction pathways associated with apoptosis induced by different types of insults to neurons (e.g., glutamate and free radicals). It will also be important to determine if the various criteria for apoptosis outlined above occur as a consequence of each of these transduction pathways or are associated predominantly with one pathway over another.

References

Ankarcrona M., Dypbukt J. M., Bonfoco E., Zhivotovsky B., Orrenius S., Lipton S. A., and Nicotera P. (1995) Glutamate-induced neuronal death: a succession of necrosis or apoptosis depending on mitochondrial function. *Neuron* **15,** 961–973.

Arends M. J. and Wyllie A. H. (1991) Apoptosis: mechanisms and roles in pathology. *Int. Rev. Exp. Pathol.* **32,** 223–254.

Bonfoco E., Krainc D., Ankarcrona M., Nicotera P., and Lipton S. A. (1995) Apoptosis and necrosis: two distinct events induced, respectively, by mild and intense insults with N-methyl-D-aspartate or nitric oxide/superoxide in cortical cell cultures. *Proc. Natl. Acad. Sci. USA* **92,** 7162–7166.

Brown D. G., Sun X.-M., and Cohen G. M. (1993) Dexamethasone-induced apoptosis involves cleavage of DNA to large fragments prior to internucleosomal fragmentation. *J. Biol. Chem.* **268,** 3037–3039.

Deckwerth T. L. and Johnson E. M., Jr. (1994) Neurites can remain viable after destruction of the neuronal soma by programmed cell death (apoptosis). *Dev. Biol.* **165,** 63–72.

Gavrieli Y., Sherman Y., and Ben-Sasson S. A. (1992) Identification of programmed cell death *in situ* via specific labeling of nuclear DNA fragmentation. *J. Cell. Biol.* **119,** 493–501.

Lipton S. A. and Rosenberg P. A. (1994) Mechanisms of disease: excitatory amino acids as a final common pathway for neurologic disorders. *New Engl. J. Med.* **330,** 613–622.

Oberhammer F., Wilson J. W., Dive C., Morris I. D., Hickman J. A., Wakeling A. E., Walker P. R., and Sikorska M. (1993) Apoptotic death in epithelial cells: cleavage of DNA to 300 and/or 50 kb fragments prior to or in the absence of internucleosomal fragmentation. *EMBO J.* **12,** 3679–3684.

Wyllie A. H. (1980) Glucocorticoid–induced thymocyte apoptosis is associated with endogenous endonuclease activation. *Nature* **284,** 555,556.

Yun J. and Kenney R. A. (1976) Preparation of cat kidney for ultrastructural studies. *J. Electron Microsc.* (Tokyo) **25,** 11–23.

Zhivotovsky B., Wade D., Gahm A., Orrenius S., and Nicotera P. (1994) Formation of 50 kbp chromatin fragments in isolated liver nuclei is mediated by protease and endonuclease activation. *FEBS Lett.* **351,** 150–154.

The Nematode
Caenorhabditis elegans
as a Model System
to Study Neuronal Cell Death

Paul Desjardins and Stéphane Ledoux

1. Introduction

Normal development and homeostasis result from a tenuous balance between cell proliferation and cell death. Disruption of this balance, in favor of cell death in particular, could easily lead to pathological states in postmitotic organs such as the adult brain (*see* Thompson, 1995). For example, many neurodegenerative disorders are characterized by the premature death of specific subsets of neurons, which gives rise to their full clinical spectra (Coleman and Flood, 1987; Choi, 1988). Although a complete understanding of the selective cell degeneration in these conditions is still lacking, recent observations suggest that it may occur through apoptosis, a gene-directed type of cell death (Bredesen, 1995). In many cases, cell death by apoptosis requires an active role by the dying cells, because apoptosis is most often significantly blocked or delayed by inhibitors of RNA or protein synthesis (Wyllie et al., 1984). This genetic regulation of apoptosis offers a potential for therapeutic intervention and further assessment of apoptotic mechanisms in manifestations of neuropathology is warranted. However, employing conventional molecular and biochemical approaches, attempts to determine the genetic machinery

From: *Neuromethods, Vol. 29: Apoptosis Techniques and Protocols*
Ed: J. Poirier Humana Press Inc.

responsible for specifying which cells live and which cells die have not always been successful in vertebrate systems.

One organism in which programmed cell death (PCD), a physiological counterpart of apoptosis, has been extensively examined is the nematode *Caenorhabditis elegans*. Pioneering studies by Horvitz and his colleagues have unraveled the molecular cascade mediating PCD in *C. elegans* (reviewed by Ellis et al., 1991a). Genetic analysis has led to the identification of specific loci which control and execute each of the different stages of the *C. elegans* PCD pathway. Interestingly, many of these loci have been conserved during evolution and mammalian homologs of the *C. elegans* cell death genes are currently being isolated. The objective of this chapter is to underline the value of utilizing such "simple" genetic material as wild-type or mutated nematodes to increase our knowledge of such a "complex" problem as apoptosis in higher vertebrates. It is beyond our scope to give detailed protocols for basic care and maintenance of worms as well as transgenic animal construction, but references in which these can be obtained are provided in the text. Rather, we will describe the morphology and genetic pathway for PCD that normally occurs during *C. elegans* development, with an emphasis on limits and advantages of this model. Recent advances in identifying and characterizing the genes and their homologs that are critical in this process will be summarized. Next, we will outline broad strategies and methods that could be used to find additional homologous genes in other experimental systems. Finally, implications of these studies for both the understanding and prevention of neuronal cell death occurring in certain human neurological disorders will be addressed.

2. *C. elegans* as a Model System

Caenorhabditis elegans is a small nematode about 1.5 mm in length with an hermaphrodite mode of reproduction. It has a short life cycle of 3 d, and it lives for approx 17 d after reaching adulthood. In the laboratory, *C. elegans is* easily cultured on agar plates that have been overlayed with *Escherichia coli* as a food source. Readers interested in recipes for strain maintenance can be referred to Driscoll (1995). Because the living animal is transparent throughout its life cycle, its development can be directly observed at the single-cell level by light microscopy. This feature has resulted in systematic description of the cellular anatomy and cell lineage of *C. elegans* from zygote to adult (Sulston et al., 1983). In hermaphrodites, the 302 neurons and 56 glial cells account for 37% of the somatic nuclei and the entire circuitry of the nervous system has been established (Chalfie and White, 1988). Morphological analysis has also revealed that 131 of the 1090 somatic cells generated during development of an adult hermaphrodite are spatiotemporally committed or programmed to die. The whole process is generally completed within an hour of a cell's birth. This predetermined cell fate remains constant from one animal to another, that is, the same set of cells always die at the same point in development. Neurons constitute the predominant cell type to undergo these invariant changes, representing one-fifth of the entire neuronal population and approx 80% of the PCD (Horvitz et al., 1982). Mutants defective in different aspects of cell death can be readily obtained from these wild-type preparations by chemical mutagenesis (ethyl methane-sulfonate; Brenner, 1974) or exposure to ionizing radiation. Mutant phenotypes have been selected by direct observation under the dissecting microscope (10–50×), looking for morphological and behavioral defects (described by Horvitz, 1988).

The *C. elegans* haploid genome has a size of 8×10^7 nucleotide base pairs, about five times that of the yeast *Saccharomyces cerevisiae* or one fortieth that of the human genome (Waterston and Sulston, 1995). This DNA is organized into 6 nuclear chromosomes (5 autosomes and 1 X chromosome). The small nematode genome size has made increasingly refined genetic manipulations possible, allowing the cloning and molecular analysis of mutated cell death genes. These techniques are facilitated by the existence of a genetic and physical map of the *C. elegans* genome. Each chromosome is almost completely represented within an overlapping collection of cosmid (17,500) or yeast artificial clones (3500) containing well-defined genetic loci. About 22.5 Mb of the genome has been sequenced at the present time and 45% of the 4255 putative protein coding genes have significant similarity to non-*C. elegans* genes. The self-fertilizing nature of the animal permits heterozygous recessive mutations to be automatically segregated as homozygotes in the self-progeny, eliminating the need for genetic crosses. In addition, this ability of hermaphrodites makes generally lethal mutations in other systems (because of severe behavioral and anatomical defects) viable in *C. elegans* Finally, the feasibility of introducing nucleic acids into *C. elegans* oocytes by microinjection permits transgenic nematodes to be constructed, providing in vivo models to examine the activities of selected genes (Mello et al., 1992). Thus, despite some restrictions such as the lack of a cell culture system and the rapidity of the cell death process itself, the simplicity of this animal, transparency, ease of cultivation, as well as its rapid life cycle and small genome size give *C. elegans* distinct advantages as an experimental system for neuronal cell death studies.

3. Programmed Cell Death in *C. elegans*

3.1. Morphological Analysis

Identification of PCD in *C. elegans* has been based primarily on morphological studies of dying cells *in situ* using both light (100X) and electron microscopy. Most data acquisition in these studies are usually supported by Nomarski differential interference contrast (DIC) optics. This optical system amplifies differences in the refractive indices of different cellular components, facilitating precise nuclear description. The descriptive exactness of the cell death mutant can also be improved by fixation and staining with vital dyes (Hoechst 33258, diamidinophenylindole [DAPI]), or by working in a genetic background in which cell corpse phagocytosis is deficient. Repeated observations have revealed the existence of five distinct stages during the course of *C. elegans*

PCD, each characterized by discrete morphological changes (reviewed by Driscoll, 1992). Some of these morphological features are reminiscent of a cell death process, commonly found in other invertebrates and vertebrates, termed apoptosis (reviewed by Wyllie et al., 1980). The similarities include membrane blebbing, condensation of the cytoplasm and nuclear chromatin, formation of apoptotic bodies and phagocytosis by neighboring cells. These ultrastructural changes can be distinguished from the ones seen in another form of cell death termed necrosis or oncosis, in which cells undergo membrane disruption, cellular swelling, and lysis followed by the initiation of an inflammatory process (Majno and Joris, 1995). Necrosis, in a specific genetic background, can also occur in C. *elegans*. This type of cell death can be induced by mutations in a novel gene family called degenerins, perhaps encoding subunits of a cation channel complex (Chalfie and Wolinski, 1990; Driscoll and Chalfie, 1991; Canessa et al., 1993). However, because of editorial constraints, this subject will be only briefly discussed in Section 6. of this chapter.

3.2. Genetic Analysis

Systematic genetic studies in C. *elegans* have identified a large number of mutations that interfere with a four-step PCD pathway that includes the decision to die, the execution of cell death, the engulfment of cell corpses, and the degradation of chromatin. So far, 14 genes that participate in this genetic pathway have been defined (Ellis et al., 1991a). Two autosomal recessive death effector genes, *ced-3* and *ced-4* (*cell death* abnormal) are responsible for the execution of the death sentence. Somatic cells usually committed to die in *ced-3* or *ced-4* mutants survive, differentiate, and function normally, suggesting that PCD is not essential for viability of C. *elegans*. Genetic mosaic experiments have revealed that *ced-3* and *ced-4* act autonomously within the dying cells either directly by producing cytotoxic products or indirectly by controlling the activities of cytotoxic proteins (Yuan and Horvitz, 1990). One autosomal dominant gene, *ced-9*, negatively regulates PCD, acting in parallel to *ced-3* and *ced-4* in the suicide program.

The function of *ced-9 is* to protect cells that should survive from undergoing PCD. Mutations that inactivate *ced-9* are lethal for the embryo (Hengartner et al., 1992). Six other genes (*ced-1, ced-2, ced-5, ced-6, ced-7,* and *ced-10)* are necessary for the engulfment of cell corpses. None of these mutations completely block phagocytosis, suggesting the existence of more than one biochemical pathway for the elimination of cell corpses (Ellis et al., 1991b). Finally, the *nuc-1* (*nuc*lease) gene is required for the degradation of the chromatin in dying cells (Hevelone and Hartman, 1988). However, PCD proceeds normally in *nuc-1* mutant nematodes, except that the DNA of dying cells remains in pyknotic bodies. This observation indicates that *nuc-1* activity is not required for the initiation of cell death or phagocytosis, and, an as yet unidentified nuclease essential for killing cells may exist in C. *elegans.*

In addition to the C. *elegans* genes intrinsically acting in the death process, mutational analysis has revealed the existence of three genes, *ces-1 (c*ell death specification), *ces-2,* and *egl-1 (e*gg-laying abnormal) that disrupt the death-vs-life decision of specific group of cells (serotonergic NSM and HSN neurons) (Ellis and Horvitz, 1991). These results suggest that activation of the cell death pathway may be regulated by the expression of cell-specific genes, and that many more genes of this class likely exist.

3.3. Molecular Analysis

Molecular cloning of some of the *ced* genes was achieved by a combination of genetic mapping of restriction fragment length polymorphisms, transposon tagging, and construction of transgenic animals. Generally, candidate cosmids were microinjected into the mitotic germline of *ced* mutants and tested for their ability to rescue the phenotype. Characterization of these genes has revealed many exciting findings. The *ced-3* gene encodes a 503 amino acid putative protein homologous to the mammalian cysteine protease interleukin-1β (IL-1β) converting enzyme (ICE) (Yuan et al., 1993). This finding suggests that the execution of PCD in C. *elegans* is mediated by protease activity, and that ICE may control apoptosis in vertebrates. The *ced-4* gene encodes a novel hydrophilic protein of 549 amino acids with no obvious transmembrane domain (Yuan and Horvitz, 1992). The CED-4 protein has no significant similarity to other known polypeptides. The presence of two regions in the CED-4 sequence with EF-hand calcium-binding motif initially led to the suggestion that its activity was regulated by divalent cations, but the significance of this latter observation has been recently questioned (Horvitz et al., 1994). *Ced-3* and *ced-4* are predominantly expressed during embryogenesis, when most PCD takes place in *C. elegans*. Molecular characterization of the *C. elegans ced-9* repressor gene has shown that it encodes an inferred 280 amino acid protein homologous to the mammalian *bcl-2* proto-oncogene product (Hengartner and Horvitz, 1994).

4. Characterization of *ced* Homologs in Vertebrate Systems

4.1. Positive Regulators of Programmed Cell Death

As already mentioned, the *ced-3* gene encodes a protein homologous to the human ICE. In mammalian cells, ICE is required for conversion of the 33 kDa inactive form of IL-1β into its 17.5 kDa active form, by cleaving after Asp residues (Cerretti et al., 1992). Overexpression of ICE in fibroblasts induces apoptosis (Miura et al., 1993). This observation suggests that ICE, or a related cysteine protease, mediates mammalian cell death. This hypothesis is supported by the fact that microinjection of crmA, a protein inhibitor of ICE, can block apoptotic cell death of chick dorsal root ganglion cells in response to growth factor deprivation (Gagliardini et al., 1994). Additional members of the *ced-3/ice* gene family have been cloned during the last two years. Some homologs were simply cloned by direct screening of cDNA libraries with an ICE coding sequence. Others were isolated by a combination of reverse transcription and low stringency polymerase chain reaction (PCR) using degenerate oligonucleotides encoding a conserved pentameric motif (QACRG) that encompasses the catalytic site of CED-3/ICE. The actual list

Table 1
Protein Sequence Homology
Among *ced*-Related Modulators of Apoptosis

CED-3-related	% Identity	% Similarity	Effect on apoptosis
ICE	29%	54%	proapoptotic
ICE_{rel}-II/ICH-2/TX	26%	51%	proapoptotic
ICE_{rel}-III	25%	51%	proapoptotic
$ICH-1_L$	28%	52%	proapoptotic
$ICH-1_S$	27%	52%	antiapoptotic
CPP32/Yama/Apopain	35%	58%	proapoptotic
Mch2	35%	55%	proapoptotic
Mch3	33%	54%	proapoptotic
NEDD-2	31%	54%	proapoptotic

CED-9-related	% Identity	% Similarity	Effect on apoptosis
Bcl-2	23%	46%	antiapoptotic
$Bcl-X_L$	20%	46%	antiapoptotic
$Bcl-X_S$	18%	45%	proapoptotic
Bax	18%	50%	proapoptotic
Bak	23%	53%	proapoptotic
Bad	17%	42%	proapoptotic
MCL-1	25%	50%	antiapoptotic

The CED-3 and CED-9 sequences are compared to the protein sequence database provided by the National Center for Biotechnology Information (NCBI) using the Bestfit algorithm.

of CED-3 homologs (depicted in Table 1a) includes human ICE_{rel}-II/TX/ICH-2 (Faucheu et al., 1995; Kamens et al., 1995; Munday et al., 1995), ICE_{rel}-III (Munday et al., 1995), CPP32/Yama/Apopain (Fernandes-Alnemri et al., 1994), Mch-2 (Fernandes-Alnemri et al., 1995a), Mch-3 (Fernandes-Alnemri et al., 1995b), ICH-1 (Wang et al., 1994), and a murine homolog, NEDD-2 (Kumar et al., 1994). Their expression is partly regulated by alternative splicing and they have a proenzymatic organization. As with ICE, ectopic expression of these proteases causes apoptosis. Since overexpression of practically any protease in cells is likely to provoke cell death (Williams and Henkart, 1994), and since some cell lines that do not express detectable levels of ICE can undergo apoptosis (Ceretti et al., 1992), it remains to be determined which member(s) of this cysteine protease family play a decisive role in mammalian PCD. Furthermore, recent studies on ICE knockout mice suggest that ICE itself is not always a prerequisite for apoptosis initiation (Kuida et al., 1995; Li et al., 1995).

One tool that could further elucidate this controversy has been recently developed. In an attempt to improve our understanding of the biochemistry during the active phase of apoptosis, Lazebnik et al. have developed a powerful system based on a cell-free extract (1993). Briefly, this cell-free system is made from cytosolic preparations obtained from chicken hepatoma cells that have been blocked sequentially in S-phase with aphidicolin for 12 h, and subsequently in M-phase with nocodazole for 3 h. Mitotic cells are then harvested by selective detachment (mitotic shake-off), washed, and lysed in a Dounce homogenizer after several cycles of freezing and thawing. The cell lysate (the S/M extract) is then centrifuged for 3 h at 150,000g to yield a clear supernatant. When added to isolated HeLa nuclei, this cell-free extract reproduces the morphological changes observed during apoptosis. With this death extract, the authors have shown the cleavage of the nuclear enzyme poly (ADP-ribose) polymerase (PARP) (Lazebnik et al., 1994). PARP is usually involved in DNA repair, genome surveillance and integrity (Schreiber et al., 1995). It is one of the proteins known to be cleaved in association with apoptosis (Kaufman et al., 1993). Inhibitors and cleavage site studies eventually led to the hypothesis that the enzyme responsible for PARP proteolytic cleavage was similar but distinct from ICE. This enzyme was termed prICE (*p*rotease *r*esembling ICE) and the encoding gene has been cloned almost simultaneously by two different groups. This cysteine protease was called Yama (Tewari et al., 1995) or Apopain (Nicholson et al., 1995) and sequence analysis has revealed that it is identical to the product of the *CPP32* gene (Fernandes-Alnemri et al., 1994), another CED-3-like molecule. Other substrates such as the 70 kDa protein component of the U1 small nuclear ribonucleoprotein, lamin B1, α-fodrin, topoisomerase I, and β-actin (Martin and Green, 1995) are also targeted by proteases during apoptosis and the same cell-free extract paradigm could be used to try to pinpoint the offender.

4.2. Negative Regulators of Programmed Cell Death

As seen previously, the *ced-9* repressor gene encodes an inferred protein with sequence and structural similarities to the product of the mammalian *bcl-2* proto-oncogene (Hengartner and Horvitz, 1994). *Bcl-2* was initially identified as part of a chromosomal rearrangement in follicular B-cell lymphomas (Cleary et al., 1986). Bcl-2 is an inner mitochondrial membrane protein that negatively regulates PCD when overexpressed in mammalian cells (Hockenbery et al., 1990). Interestingly, expression of the human *bcl-2* in nematodes partially suppress programmed cell deaths, suggesting an evolutionarily conserved function (Vaux et al., 1992; Hengartner and Horvitz, 1994).

New studies in mammals have revealed the existence of an emerging family of CED-9/Bcl-2-related proteins (Table 1b). This family now includes Bax (Oltvai et al., 1993), Bak (Chittenden et al., 1995; Farrow et al., 1995; Kiefer et al., 1995), Bcl-x (Boise et al., 1993; Gonzalez-Garcia et al., 1994), MCL1 (Kozopas et al., 1993) and murine Bad (Yang et al., 1995). Although their percentages of identity with the Ced-9 protein are <25%, all these Bcl-2-related proteins share two highly conserved domains termed BH1 and BH2 (*Bcl-2 Homology*) which constitute novel dimerization motifs (Yin et al., 1994). Various strategies were employed to characterize these additional *ced-9/bcl-2* family gene members. One of them, *bcl-x* was initially found by screening a chicken cDNA library under low stringency conditions with a murine *bcl-2* cDNA probe. Chicken *bcl-x* was subsequently used to isolate two distinct cDNAs derived from alternative splicing of the human *bcl-x* gene: *bcl-x$_L$* and *bcl-x$_S$*. *Bcl-x$_L$*, the longest isoform, encodes a protein that inhibits cell death. Paradoxically, the other transcript, *bcl-x$_S$*, produces a protein that antagonizes the protective action of Bcl-2 by an unknown mechanism. Another Bcl-2-related protein, Bad, has been cloned using the yeast two-hybrids system, after a screening for proteins that interact with Bcl-2. As for Bax, it was initially identified by coimmunoprecipitation as a 21 kDa Bcl-2-associated protein. Bax cDNA was then obtained after microsequencing the purified peptide and designing a degenerate oligonucleotide to probe a cDNA library. Finally, Bak was cloned by screening cDNA libraries with PCR primers based on degenerate oligonucleotides encoding the BH1 and BH2 conserved domains. Like Bcl-x_s, Bax, Bad, and Bak promote PCD. Taken together, these findings demonstrate that the apoptotic process is tightly regulated by a complex network of interactions among members of the *ced-9/bcl-2* gene family, superimposed on proapoptotic influences from the *ced-3/ice* gene family.

5. Isolation of Additional *ced* Homologs in Vertebrate Systems

5.1. General Comment

Data presented in the previous sections on the involvement of the *ced-3/ice* and *ced-9/bcl-2* gene families in both nematode and vertebrate apoptosis strongly support the idea that cell death mechanisms are phylogenetically conserved. These data also suggest that perhaps other genes implicated in *C. elegans* PCD have equivalents in mammalian systems, and create interesting experimental opportunities for a better understanding of neuronal apoptosis. Among other things, the availability of additional *ced* gene sequences in the near future may provide the means to identify novel homologs in other species. With this eventuality in mind, we will now discuss some general strategies and methods (illustrated in Fig. 1) that could be used to isolate vertebrate homologs of the *C. elegans* PCD cascade when DNA sequence and protein databases do not yield significant homology.

5.2. Low Stringency Hybridization

One of the first steps in the isolation of other members of a putative gene family consists of using low stringency hybridization with genomic DNA from different branches of the phylogenetic tree (zoo blot). The reasoning for this type

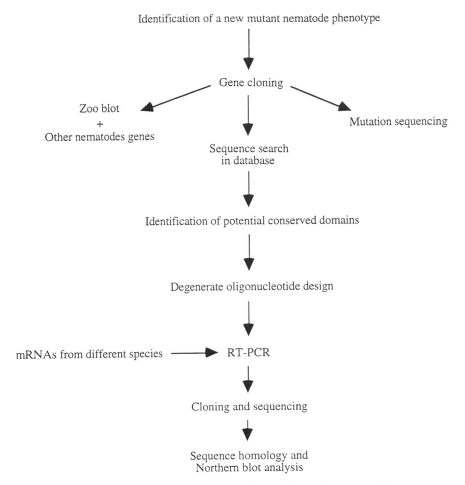

Fig. 1. Strategies for cloning vertebrate homologs of *ced* gene.

of approach is twofold. First of all, it gives us a rapid survey of which organism is likely to have homology For example, crosshybridizing DNA sequences from *mec-4* have been detected in vertebrates, leading to the prediction that it was part of a larger family (Driscoll and Chalfie, 1991). The recent cloning in rat distal colon of an epithelial sodium channel sharing significant similarity with *mec-4* proved that was the case. (Canessa et al., 1993). Secondly, identifying a positive or negative signal in other systems with cDNA probes from different portions of the gene, may help to define which domains of the encoded protein are likely to be of functional importance. This strategy has led to the successful identification of a new member of the MyoD gene family (Michelson et al., 1990). The genomic DNA to be probed should be extracted from a broad variety of species. Indeed, going directly from *C. elegans* to mammals by nucleic acid hybridization may give false-negative results. Instead, it is more productive to climb progressively up the evolutionary tree by looking at organisms more closely related to *C. elegans (S. cerevisiae*, tunicate, *D. melanogaster*, sea urchin, and so on). Moreover, cloning and sequencing of additional homologs from related nematode species (*C. briggsae, C. vulgariensis*, and so on) as well as mutation characterization could increase the ability to determine conserved regions of the gene.

5.2.1. Procedure

1. Prepare DNAs from different sources.
2. Genomic DNAs are digested with restriction enzymes (*Eco*RI, *Hind*III, and so on), electrophoresed on 0.7% agarose gels, and transferred to nitrocellulose as described (Maniatis et al., 1982).
3. Hybridize with a ^{32}P-labeled probe synthesized by random priming from the entire cDNA of interest. The conditions for hybridization are 6X SSC, 5X Denhardt's reagent, 100 μg/mL salmon sperm DNA, 1 mM EDTA, 10 mM sodium phosphate buffer, pH 7.0, and 0.5% SDS. Hybridization is carried out at 45°C for a minimum of 18 h.
4. Filters are washed in 2X SSC and 0.5% SDS at 37, 45, and 50°C, successively. Expose overnight.
5. Different cDNAs subfragments can be evaluated to assess which portion is responsible for homology, if the initial screening is positive.

5.3. Cloning of Homologs
by Reverse Transcription-Polymerase Chain Reaction

Reverse transcription-polymerase chain reaction (RT-PCR), an experimental method to clone putative members of a novel gene family, was adopted for the identification of odorant receptors by Buck and Axel (1991). The advantages of this procedure are that it necessitates only a minimal amount of total RNA and does not need the construction of cDNA libraries. However, the number of false-positives is high and criteria to decide which clone to analyze further must be developed (*see* Section 5.4.).

5.3.1. Comment

It would be of interest to use both embryonic and adult tissues as a source of total RNA. Indeed, apoptotic cell death genes should be mostly expressed during development, and comparison of amplified products from different developmental stages could give an indication regarding which band should be cloned and analyzed further. A similar strategy, using a differential screening approach, has been successful in cloning a developmentally regulated *ced* homolog in mouse (Kumar et al., 1992).

5.3.2. Degenerate Oligonucleotides Design

Degenerate oligonucleotides necessary for the RT-PCR should be designed according to the most likely conserved regions identified by zoo blot, cloning of related nematode genes, and mutation analysis. Primers separated by <500 nucleotides should be chosen, based on the estimated size of the homology Indeed, the efficacy of Taq DNA polymerase is increased with relatively short amplified products and their sequences can be analyzed more quickly.

5.3.3. Procedure

1. Total RNA (1 µg) is mixed with 10 mM Tris-HCl, pH 8.3, 1.5 mM MgCl$_2$, 50 mM KCl, 0.01% (w/v) gelatin, 200 µM dNTPs, primers at 1 µM each, AMV reverse transcriptase (80 U/mL), Taq DNA polymerase (50 U/mL) and 0.5 µCi [^{32}P]α-dATP (3000 Ci/mmol), for a total reaction volume of 50 µL, and overlaid with 100 µL of mineral oil.
2. The samples are placed in a thermal cycler at 50°C for 10 min followed by PCR at 94°C for 30 s. 40°C for 1 min, and 72°C for 1 min for 30 cycles. Different annealing temperatures should be tested.

3. The samples are electrophoresed on a low melting agarose gel.
4. DNA band(s) of the targeted size are ligated to a
   Bluescript plasmid that has been previously T-tailed
   (Marchuk et al., 1990). Briefly, this vector is prepared by
   digestion with *Eco*RV and incubation with Taq DNA
   polymerase (1 U/μg plasmid/20 μL volume) using standard buffer conditions in the presence of 2 m*M* dTTP
   for 2 h at 70°C. Ligation is done at 14°C.

5.4. Sequencing and Data Analysis

DNA sequences can be determined using the Sequenase
kit (US Biochemicals, Cleveland, OH) and protocols can be
obtained from the manufacturer.

Several computer programs can be utilized to analyze
the amplified product sequences. For example, Bestfit will
compare the obtained sequence with the one from the paren-
tal gene (Devereux et al., 1984). The Tfasta program, on the
other hand, will challenge the same sequence of interest at
the protein level after translating the nucleotide sequence for
all the six reading frames (Devereux et al., 1984). Some criteria can be introduced to orient the investigator about which
clones could be more promising, since low stringency PCR
is known to generate false-priming artifacts. One method
consists of enriching the DNA sequences by performing a
secondary amplification with nested primers (Fernandes-
Alnemri, 1995a). In addition, the final PCR product should
contain both the forward and the reverse primers and the
whole sequence should be in the right orientation.

6. Implications of Programmed Cell Death Studies in *C. elegans* for Neuronal Cell Death and Human Neurological Disorders

The possibility that apoptotic genes may play an important role in neurological diseases is frequently raised. Although
50% or more of neurons die by apoptosis during normal
development of the vertebrate nervous system, clear evidence

for dysregulation of this type of cell death has never been shown in neuropathology (Bredesen, 1995). However, experimental tools derived from the *C. elegans* model and molecular analysis of the *ced* genes and their homologs are already contributing to our attempt to validate this hypothesis. For example, morphological and biochemical features of apoptosis can be reproduced in vitro or in vivo by exposing neuronal cells to a variety of insults such as growth factor deprivation, oxidative stress or toxic agents (Thompson, 1995). Some of the neuronal death induced by these stimuli can be suppressed, both in vitro and in vivo, using specific peptide inhibitors that block the proteolytic activity of the ICE family (Milligan et al., 1995). Similarly, expression of Bcl-2 inhibits the neuronal cell death induced by NGF removal, exposition to calcium ionophores, glutamate, and β-amyloid (Bredesen, 1995), and it reduces the size of cerebral infarct in transgenic mice overexpressing *bcl-2* (Martinou et al., 1994). These findings suggest that apoptosis is mediated by a common pathway conserved through phylogeny, and the extension of these to pathological conditions is warranted.

Another potentially fruitful avenue provided by the *C. elegans* model is the use of cell death mutants or transgenic nematodes. For example, mutations in the *C. elegans deg*-1 and *mec*-4 genes cause late onset degeneration of a restricted number of neurons, and these degenerative phenotypes display a dominant inheritance pattern sometimes encountered in familial Alzheimer's disease (AD) (Driscoll, 1992). These mutants show vacuolization and lysis of neuronal cells involved in touch reception circuitry, although the viability of the animal is not threatened. More recently, the development of a transgenic *C. elegans* model expressing β-amyloid protein (βA) has been reported in the literature (Link, 1995). β-amyloid deposits in senile plaques of AD brains constitute one of the pathological hallmarks of the disease, and mutations in its βA precursor gene account for 5% of familial presenile AD (Goate et al., 1991). Interestingly, recent data have revealed that cultured neurons exposed to a synthetic β-amyloid peptide are probably undergoing apoptosis (Loo et al.,

1993). Such approaches could help in the elucidation of the normal and abnormal biological functions of molecules related to the pathogenesis of neurodegenerative diseases and in the development of novel therapeutic interventions.

7. Summary and Future Prospects

The extensive characterization of C. *elegans* PCD already contributes to our understanding of the control and mechanism of mammalian apoptosis. The biological significance of two large gene families has been revealed by the cloning of *ced-3* and *ced-9*. Results suggest a conservation of basic cell death molecular events during evolution, although a higher level of complexity has been gained in vertebrates. However, several *ced* genes remain to be identified, mapped, and analyzed, and mammalian homolog(s) of *ced-4* have not yet been found. As well, further experiments are needed to determine how the CED-9/Bcl-2 family members suppress the action of the CED3/ICE family members. Utilization of actual and future resources in the PCD field will hopefully address these issues.

Acknowledgments

We would like to thank Josephine Nalbantoglu and Junying Yuan for critical reading of the manuscript. We appreciate the technical assistance of Jean-Pascal de Waele. This work is supported by the Fondation de l'hôpital St-Luc.

References

Boise L. H., González-Garcia M., Postema C. E., Ding L., Lindsten T., Turka L. A., Mao X., Nunez G., and Thompson C. B. (1993) *bcl-x*, a *bcl*-2-related gene that functions as a dominant regulator of apoptic cell death. *Cell* **74**, 597–608.

Bredesen D. E. (1995) Neural apoptosis. *Ann. Neurol.* **38**, 839–851.

Brenner S. (1974) The genetics of *Caenorhabditis elegans*. *Genetics* **77**, 71–94.

Buck L. and Axel R. (1991) A novel multigene family may encode odorant receptors: a molecular basis for odor recognition. *Cell* **65**, 175–187.

Canessa C. M., Horisberger J.-D., and Rossier B C (1993) Epithelial sodium channel related to proteins involved in neurodegeneration. *Nature* **361,** 467–470.

Cerretti D. P., Kozlosky C. J., Mosley B., Nelson N., Ness K. V., Greenstreet T. A., March C. J., Kronheim S. R., Druck T., Cannizzaro L. A., Huebner K., and Black R. A (1992) Molecular cloning of the interleukin-1β-converting enzyme *Science* **256,** 97–100.

Chalfie M. and White J. (1988) The nervous system, in *The Nematode Caenorhabditis elegans.* Cold Spring Harbor Laboratory, Cold Spring Harbor, NY.

Chalfie M. and Wolinsky E. (1990) The identification and suppression of inherited neurodegeneration in *Caenorhabditis elegans. Nature* **345,** 410–416.

Chittenden T., Harrington E. A., O'Connor R., Flemington C., Lutz R. J., Evan G. I., and Guild B. C. (1995) Induction of apoptosis by the Bcl-2 homolog Bak. *Nature* **374,** 733– 736.

Choi D. (1988) Glutamate neurotoxicity and diseases of the nervous system. *Neuron* **1,** 623–634.

Cleary M. L., Smith S. D., and Sklar J. (1986) Cloning and structural analysis of cDNAs for *bcl-2* and a hybrid *bcl-2/*immunoglobulin transcript resulting from the t(14; 18) translocation. *Cell* **47,** 19–28.

Coleman P. D. and Flood D. G. (1987) Neuron numbers and dendritic extent in normal aging and Alzheimer's disease. *Neurobiol. Aging* **8,** 521–545.

Devereux J., Haeberli P., and Smithies O. (1984) A comprehensive set of sequence analysis programs. *Nucleic Acids Res.* **12,** 387–395.

Driscoll M. and Chalfie M. (1991) The *mec-4* gene is a member of a family of *Caenorhabditis elegans* genes that can mutate to induce neuronal degeneration. *Nature* **349,** 588–593.

Driscoll M. (1992) Molecular genetics of cell death inthe nematode *Caenorhabditis elegans. J. Neurobiol.* **23,** 1327–1351.

Driscoll M. (1995) Methods for the study of cell death in the nematode *Caenorhabditis elegans,* in *Methods in Cell Biology,* vol. 46 (Schwartz L. M. and Osborne B. A. eds.), Academic, NY, pp. 323–353.

Ellis R. E. and Horvitz H. R. (1991) Two *C. elegans* genes control the programmed death of specific cells in the pharynx. *Development* **112,** 591–603.

Ellis R. E., Yuan J., and Horvitz H. R. (1991a) Mechanism and functions of cell death. *Ann. Rev. Cell Biol.* **7,** 663–698.

Ellis R. E., Jacobson D. M., and Horvitz H. R. (1991b) Genes required for the engulfment of cell corpses during programmed cell death in *Caenorhabditis elegans. Genetics* **129,** 79–94.

Farrow S. N., White J. H. M., Martinou I., Raven T., Pun K.-T., Grinham C. J., Martinou J.-C., and Brown R. (1995). Cloning of a *bcl-2* homologue by interaction with adenovirus E1B 19K. *Nature* **374,** 731–733.

Faucheu C., Diu A., Chan A. W. E., Blanchet A.-M., Miossec C., Herve F., Collard- Dutilleul V., Gu Y., Aldape R. A., Lippke J. A., Rocher C., Su M. S. S., Livingston D. J., Hercend T., and Lalanne J.-L. (1995). A novel human protease similar to the interleukin-1β converting enzyme induces apoptosis in transfected cells. *EMBO J.* **14,** 1914–1922.

Fernandes-Alnemri T., Litwack G., and Alnemri E. S. (1994) CPP32, a novel human apoptotic protein with homology to *Caenorhabditis elegans* cell death protein ced-3 and mammalian interleukin-1β-converting enzyme. *J. Biol. Chem.* **269,** 30,761–30,764.

Fernandes-Alnemri T., Litwack G., and Alnemri E. S. (1995a) *Mch-2,* a new member of the apoptotic *ced-3/Ice* cysteine protease gene family. *Cancer Res.* **55,** 2737–2742.

Fernandes-Alnemri T., Takahashi A., Armstrong R., Krebs J., Fritz L., Tomaselli K. J., Wang L., Yu Z., Croce C. M., Salveson G., Earnshaw W. C., Litwack G., and Alnemri E. S. (1995b) Mch3, a novel human apoptotic cysteine protease highly related to CPP32. *Cancer Res.* **55,** 6045–6052.

Gagliardini V., Fernandez P. A., Lee R. K. K., Drexler H. C. A., Rotello R. J., Fishman M., and Yuan J. (1994) Prevention of vertebrate neuronal death by the *crmA* gene. *Science* **263,** 826–828.

Goate A., Chartier–Harlin M. C., Mullan M., Brown J., Crawford F., Fidani L., Giuffra L., Haynes A., Irving N., James L. et al. (1991) Segregation of a missense mutation in the amyloid precursor protein gene with familial Alzheimer's disease. *Nature* **349,** 704–706.

González-Garcia M., Pérez-Ballestro R., Ding L., Duan L., Boise L. H., Thompson C. B., and Nunez G. (1994) *bcl-x$_L$* is the major *bcl-x* mRNA form expressed during murine development and its product localizes to mitochondria. *Development* **120,** 3033–3042.

Hengartner M. O., Ellis R. E., and Horvitz H. R. (1992) *C. elegans* gene *ced-9* protects cells from programmed cell death. *Nature* **356,** 494–499.

Hengartner M. O. and Horvitz H. R. (1994) *C. elegans* cell survival gene *ced-9* encodes a functional homolog of the mammalian proto-oncogene *bcl-2. Cell* **76,** 665–676.

Hevelone J. and Hartman P. S. (1988) An endonuclease from *Caenorhabditis elegans:* partial purification and characterization. *Biochem. Genet.* **26,** 447–461.

Hockenbery D., Nunez G., Milliman C., Schreiber R. D., and Korsmeyer S. J. (1990) Bcl-2 is an inner mitochondrial membrane protein that blocks programmed cell death. *Nature* **348,** 334–336.

Horvitz H. R., Ellis H. M., and Sternberg P. W. (1982) Programmed cell death in nematode development. *Neurosci. Comment* **1,** 56–65.

Horvitz H. R. (1988) Genetics of cell lineage, in *The Nematode Caenorhadbitis elegans.* Cold Spring Harbor Laboratory, Cold Spring Harbor, NY.

Horvitz H. R., Shaham S., and Hengartner M. O. (1994) The genetics of programmed cell death in the nematode *Caenorhabditis elegans*. *Cold Spring Harbor Symposia on Quantitative Biology,* vol. 59, pp. 377–385.

Kamens J., Paskind M., Hugunin M., Talanian R. V., Allen H., Banach D., Bump N., Hackett M., Johnston C. G., Li P., Mankovich J. A., Terranova M., and Ghayur T. (1995) Identification and characterization of ICH-2, a novel member of the interleukin-1β-converting enzyme family of cysteine proteases. *J. Biol. Chem.* **270,** 15,250–15,256.

Kaufmann S. H., Desnoyers S., Ottaviano Y., Davidson N. E., and Poirier G. G. (1993) Specific proteolytic cleavage of poly (ADP-ribose) polymerase: an early marker of chemotherapy-induced apoptosis. *Cancer Res.* **53,** 3976–3985.

Kiefer M. C., Brauer M. J., Powers V. C., Wu J. J., Umansky S. R., Tomei L. D., and Barr P. J. (1995) Modulation of apoptosis by the widely distributed Bcl-2 homolog Bak. *Nature* **374,** 736–739.

Kozopas K. M., Yang T., Buchan H. L., Zhou P., and Craig R. W. (1993) MCL1, a gene expressed in programmed myeloid cell differentiation, has sequence similarity to BCL2. *Proc. Natl. Acad. Sci. USA* **90,** 3516–3520.

Kuida K., Lippke J. A., Ku G., Harding M. W., Livingston D. J., Su M. S.-S., and Flavell R. A. (1995) Altered cytokine export and apoptosis in mice deficient in interleukin-1β converting enzyme. *Science* **267,** 2000–2003.

Kumar S., Tomooka Y., and Noda M. (1992) Identification of a set of genes with developmentally down-regulated expression in mouse brain. *Biochem. Biophys. Res. Comm.* **185,** 1155–1161.

Kumar S., Kinoshita M., Noda M., Copeland N. G., and Jenkins N. A. (1994) Induction of apoptosis by the mouse *Nedd-2* gene, which encodes a protein similar to the product of the *Caenorhabditis elegans* cell death gene *ced-3* and the mammalian IL-1β-converting enzyme. *Genes Dev.* **8,** 1613–1626.

Lazebnik Y. A., Cole S., Cooke C. A., Nelson W. G., and Earnshaw W. C. (1993) Nuclear events of apoptosis in vitro in cell-free mitotic extracts: a model system for analysis of the active phase of apoptosis. *J. Cell Biol.* **123,** 7–22.

Lazebnik Y. A., Kaufmann S. H., Desnoyers S., Poirier G. G., and Earnshaw W. C. (1994) Cleavage of poly (ADP-ribose) polymerase by a proteinase with properties like ICE. *Nature* **371,** 346,347.

Li P., Allen H., Banerjee S., Franklin S., Herzog L., Johnston C., McDowell J., Paskind M., Rodman L., Salfeld J., Towne E., Tracey D., Wardwell S., Wei F.-Y., Wong W., Kamen R., and Seshadri T. (1995) Mice deficient in IL-1β-converting enzyme are defective in production of mature IL-1β and resistant to endotoxic shock. *Cell* **80,** 401–411.

Link C. D. (1995) Expression of human β-amyloid peptide in transgenic *Caenorhabditis elegans*. *Proc. Natl. Acad. Sci. USA* **92,** 9368–9372.

Loo D. T., Copani A., Pike C. J., Whittemore E. R., Walencewicz A. J., and Cotman C. W. (1993) Apoptosis is induced by beta-amyloid in cultured central nervous system neurons. *Proc. Natl. Acad. Sci. USA* **90,** 7951–7955.

Majno G., and Joris I. (1995) Apoptosis, oncosis, and necrosis. An overview of cell death. Am. *J. Pathol.* **146,** 3–15.

Maniatis T., Fritsch E. F., and Sambrook J. (1982) *Molecular Cloning: A Laboratory Manual.* Cold Spring Harbor Laboratory, Cold Spring Harbor, NY.

Marchuk D., Drumm M., Saulino A., and Collins F. S. (1990) Construction of T-tailed vectors, a rapid and general system for direct cloning of unmodified PCR products. *Nucleic Acids Res.* **19,** 1154.

Martin S. J. and Green G. R. (1995) Protease activation during apoptosis: death by a thousand cuts? *Cell* **82,** 349–352.

Martinou J. C., Dubois-Dauphin M., Staple J. K., Rodriguez I., Frankowski H., Missoten M., Albertini P., Talabot D., Catsicas S., Pietra C., and Huarte J. (1994) Overexpression of Bcl-2 in transgenic mice protects neurons from naturally occuring cell death and experimental ischemia. *Neuron* **13,** 1017–1030.

Mello C. C., Kramer J. M., Stinchcomb D., and Ambros V. (1992) Efficient gene transfer in *C. elegans:* extrachromosomal maintenance and integration of transforming sequences. *EMBO J.* **10,** 3959–3970.

Michelson A. M., Abmayr S. M., Bate M., Arias A. M., and Maniatis T. (1990) Expression of a MyoD family member prefigures muscle pattern in *Drosophila* embryo. *Genes Dev.* **4,** 2086–2097.

Milligan C. E., Prevette D., Yaginuma H., Homma S., Cardwell C., Fritz L. C., Tomaselli K. J., Oppenheim R. W., and Schwartz L. M. (1995) Peptide inhibitors of the ICE protease family arrest programmed cell death of motoneurons *in vivo* and *in vitro. Neuron* **15,** 385–393.

Miura M., Zhu H., Rotello R., Hartwieg E. A., and Yuan J. (1993) Induction of apoptosis in fibroblast by IL-1β-converting enzyme, a mammalian homolog of the *C. elegans* cell death gene *ced-3. Cell* **75,** 653–660.

Munday N. A., Vaillancourt J. P., Ali A., Casano F. J., Miller D. K., Molineaux S. M., Yamin T.-T., Yu V. L., and Nicholson D. W. (1995) Molecular cloning and proapoptotic activity of ICE$_{rel}$- II and ICE$_{rel}$- III, members of the ICE/CED3 family of cysteine proteases. *J. Biol. Chem.* **270,** 15,870–15,876.

Nicholson D. W., Ali A., Thornberry N. A., Vaillancourt J. P., Ding C. K., Gallant M., Gareau Y., Griffin P. R., Labelle M., Lazebnik Y. A., Munday N. A., Raju S. M., Smulson M. E., Yamin T.-T., Yu V. L., and Miller D. K. (1995) Identification and inhibition of the ICE/CED-3 protease necessary for mammalian apoptosis. *Nature* **376,** 37–43.

Oltvai Z. N., Milliman C. L., and Korsmeyer S. J. (1993) Bcl-2 heterodimerizes in vivo with a conserved homolog, Bax, that accelerates programmed cell death. *Cell* **74,** 609–619.

Schreiber V., Hunting D., Trucco C., Gowans B., Grunwald D., deMurcia G., and Menissier de Murcia J. (1995) A dominant-negative mutant of human poly (ADPribose) polymerase affects cell recovery, apoptosis, and sister chromatid exchange following DNA damage. *Proc. Natl. Acad. Sci. USA* **92,** 4753–4757.

Sulston J. E. and Horvitz H. R. (1977) Postembryonic cell lineage of the nematode *Caenorhabditis elegans. Dev. Biol.* **82,** 110–156.

Sulston J. E., Schierenberg E., White J. G., and Thompson N. (1983) The embryonic cell lineage of the nematode *Caenorhabditis elegans. Dev. Biol.* **100,** 64–119.

Tewari M., Quan L. T., O'Rourke K., Desnoyers S., Zeng Z., Beidler D. R., Poirier G. G., Salvesen G. S., and Dixit V. M. (1995) Yama/CPP32β, a mammalian homolog of CED-3, is a crm-A inhibitable protease that cleaves the death substrate poly (ADP-ribose) polymerase. *Cell* **81,** 801–809.

Thompson C. B. (1995) Apoptosis in the pathogenesis and treatment of disease. *Science* **267,** 1456–1462.

Vaux D. L., Weissman I. L., and Kim S. K. (1992) Prevention of programmed cell death *in Caenorhabditis elegans* by human *bcl-2. Science* **258,** 1955–1957.

Wang L., Miura M., Bergeron L., Zhu H., and Yuan J. (1994) *Ich-1*, an *ice/ced-3-related* gene, encodes both positive and negative regulators of programmed cell death. *Cell* **78,** 739–750.

Waterston R. and Sulston J. (1995) The genome of *Caenorhabditis elegans. Proc. Natl. Acad. Sci. USA* **92,** 10,836–10,840.

Williams M. S. and Henkart P. A. (1994) Apoptotic cell death induced by intracellular proteolysis. *J. Immunol.* **153,** 4247–4255.

Wyllie A. H. (1980) Glucocorticoid-induced thymocyte apoptosis is associated with endogenous endonuclease activation. *Nature* **284,** 555,556.

Wyllie A. H., Kerr J. F. R., and Currie A. R. (1980) Cell death: the significance of apoptosis. *Intern. Rev. Cytol.* **68,** 251–306.

Wyllie A. H., Morris R. G., Smith A. L., and Dunlop D. (1984) Chromatin cleavage in apoptosis: association with condensed chromatin morphology and dependance on macromolecular synthesis. *J. Pathol.* **142,** 67–77.

Yang E., Zha J., Jockel J., Boise J. H., Thompson C. B., and Korsmeyer S. J. (1995) Bad, a heterodimeric partner for BCL-x$_L$ and Bcl-2, displaces Bax and promotes cell death. *Cell* **80,** 285–291.

Yin X.-M., Oltvai Z. N., and Korsmeyer S. T. (1994) BH1 and BH2 domains of Bcl-2 are required for inhibition of apoptosis and heterodimerization with Bax. *Nature* **369,** 321–323.

Yuan J. and Horvitz H. R. (1990) Genetic mosaic analysis of *ced-3* and *ced-4*, two genes that control programmed cell death in the nematode *C. elegans*. *Dev. Biol.* **138,** 33–41.

Yuan J. and Horvitz H. R. (1992) The *Caenorhabditis elegans* cell death gene *ced-4* encodes a novel protein and is expressed during the period of extensive programmed cell death. *Development* **116,** 309–320.

Yuan J., Shaham S., Ledoux S., Ellis H. M., and Horvitz H. R. (1993) The *C. elegans* cell death gene *ced-3* encodes a protein similar to mammalian interleukin-1β-converting enzyme. *Cell* **75,** 641–652.

Index

DATE DUE	BORROWER'S NAME	ROOM NUMBER